Ask Dr. Salk

Ask Dr. Salk

Questions and Answers
About Your Family in the 80s

❦

Dr. Lee Salk

The Bobbs-Merrill Company, Inc.
Indianapolis   New York

Portions of this book appeared in a somewhat different form in *McCall's*.

Copyright© 1981 by Dr. Lee Salk

All rights reserved, including the right of reproduction in whole or in part in any form
Published by The Bobbs-Merrill Company, Inc.
Indianapolis   New York

First printing
Library of Congress Cataloging in Publication Data

Salk, Lee, 1926 –
  Ask Dr. Salk.

  1. Children — Management. 2. Parent and child — United States. 3.
Family — United States.   4. Conduct of Life.   I. Title.
HQ769.S244   649'.1   81-66313
ISBN 0-672-52677-8   AACR2

First printing

I dedicate this book to

EGON DUMLER

*a special friend, whose faith
and optimism have been so helpful.*

My appreciation to Mary Ann O'Roark for making my work at *McCall's* Magazine so pleasant and gratifying. And to Dorothy Downie, my very special thanks not only for keeping me organized enough to get through my hectic days, but for her patience and compassion in listening to my tribulations.

Contents

CONTENTS

CONTENTS

CONTENTS

CONTENTS

CONTENTS

Introduction

The stresses on family life today are of deep concern to me. The pressures, the anguish, and the rapid bombardment caused by accelerated changes in everyday life pose a threat to the mental health of future generations. While I'm optimistic about the outcome, the ability we each have for coping with the multitude of problems we face daily depends upon our ability to remain in contact with our humanness.

While the stresses of life may be more intense today, the problems we have are basically no different from those of other times. What *is* different is that our fears and anxieties have been intensified by the mass media. Television not only brings the gory elements of death right into our living rooms, but makes us face the realities of the nuclear age. The anxiety this creates, however, is far less devastating than the desensitization it causes: we have become numb to human tragedy. It is unlikely that we will ever be able to eliminate completely the tragic outcome of human destructiveness, or that we will be able to prevent all the misfortunes we encounter in the course of life.

As a psychologist, I consider it my mission to provide insight, knowledge, and concepts that will help people cope more effectively and prevent serious problems from developing.

In this book, I address myself to the myriad problems families are facing today. I've selected a multitude of the ones heard in my consulting room that have been presented to me by a broad range of people. The information I present here is geared to help the average person deal directly with his or her own difficulties. I'm convinced that most people are capable of dealing with their problems themselves — provided they have the help of sound, practical guidance that is scientifically based. The purpose of this book is to supply precisely that.

I've addressed myself in this book to a range of matters that includes helping children develop a sense of responsibility; understanding how to cope with anger; how to respect one another's privacy; teenage rebellion; how to deal with guilt; helping children overcome fears; helping them deal with money; coping with family crises; depression; the problems of working parents; the importance of holiday traditions; the emotional aspects of physical illness; the effects of an unhappy marriage and/or divorce on children; as well as what, when, and how to tell your children about sexual matters.

I've specifically used real questions presented to me by real persons with real problems. By dealing with the specifics of what troubled them, I can focus not only on the elements of the problems themselves but on the procedures for dealing with problems of a similar nature which each person can apply to his or her own particular case.

There is absolutely no way a parent can get from one aay to another without experiencing problems. There's no such thing as having family responsibilities or being responsible for raising children without encountering paradoxical situations all along the way. Most parents at some time or other feel that only *they* are overwhelmed and unable to cope. As reassuring as this may sound to you, it doesn't diminish parental anguish, nor does it diminish the feeling that it's all too much for you to handle. Nevertheless, by sharing the experiences other people have put to me in the form of their problems, it is my hope that you not only will be more effective in dealing with problems but you will also realize that you're not alone.

In my years of practice as a psychologist, I've learned that every destructive or violent act committed by one human against another can be traced to things that happened in that person's early development. Interestingly enough, when we hear of a serious crime, a murder, or an assassination attempt, we immediately become curious about the early life of the person who's committed the act. Journalists immediately probe into the person's early behavior, performance at school, and position in the community to find an explanation or to find out what went wrong.

The family is the key social unit within which human beings learn a sense of self-esteem and develop the skills for being able to cope with life's problems later on. Only through feeling important to at least one person in the course of early growth and development can a human being learn to love — and to gain a sense of self-worth sufficient to become a useful member of society. I have no doubts that people who have felt loved during early life are far more capable of loving others in adulthood, while those who experienced emotional neglect will learn not to trust, will have difficulty expressing love, and will be vulnerable to other emotional problems.

The major problem facing families today is that they seem to have less and less time to spend with one another, and have in a sense defaulted in the responsibilities that were once a family matter. With far less parental time available to children, schools have been expected to provide the main structure in a child's life — as well as his discipline and punishment. With the little time families *do* have together, many of them spend an inordinate amount of it in front of a television screen. In this way, human, moral, and social values are heavily influenced by the material on the screen. And since more parents work today, and there's such reliance on the one-way communication that takes place with a television set, there is less opportunity for the kind of talking, listening, and human responsiveness that is essential to the nurturance of positive human qualities.

In spite of all the stresses and the negative elements in modern life, I believe this is a fascinating time to be alive. There is greater openness and honesty about life. Subjects that were totally taboo, even ten or fifteen years ago, are now often dealt with directly and matter-of-factly. Years ago, for instance, not only was pregnancy an unmentionable topic in polite conversation, but pregnant women avoided being seen in public during the advanced part of their pregnancy. Today, we no longer treat pregnancy as an illness, and we also accept the curiosity of children and their questions about reproduction. The women's movement has helped raise the consciousness of all of us, and has directed us to reexamine traditional male and traditional female roles. This has not only given women the opportunity for more options than were available twenty years ago: it has served to let men be more involved in rearing children, and to give them a more active share in household responsibilities.

I hope that in the pages ahead you will become more sensitized to what you can do to deal with the frustrations of everyday life. You will become aware of my emphasis on how important it is for family members to talk and listen to one another. A common complaint presented to me by children these days is, "My mother and father are too busy to listen to me." I urge people to use the time they spend with one another in a psychologically useful manner. Mealtime is incredibly important: it should be a time when everyone talks and listens, expresses interests and frustrations, and cooperates in making family decisions. If family mealtime is combined with television-watching, it becomes a tragic loss to a potentially useful family experience.

The pressures of life today cause parents to push their children into many responsibilities before they're ready for them. In our culture, we have a very low regard for emotional dependency. We sometimes force our children to "go out there" and deal with life's problems — without any help from us. To need assistance is viewed as a weakness. But by forcing our children to be independent before they're ready, we have in many ways weakened their capacity to form close relationships in which there is mutual dependency.

With more and more children living in single-parent households, we've had to reevaluate the consequences of the changing shape of the American family. I think we have put too much emphasis on the structure of the family and too little on the way family members relate to one another. My experience tells me that many two-parent families are not really functioning as families, despite their being structured as the "traditional" family. Such a "traditional" family often consists of nothing more than a group of people living under the same roof but where there's little interaction. Having two parents who simultaneously ignore their children provides far less gratification than single parents who spend time with their children and where there's a strong feeling of importance of each for the other in their day-to-day life.

I truly believe that we must look upon family life as being so important that people should not take on the responsibilities of being parents unless they're able to be actively involved in raising their children.

In my professional practice, I've found that many parents who have little time to spend with their children feel guilty about not providing the kind of parental contact their children need. Most people recognize the shortcomings of any substitute for a strong, meaningful, caring relationship with at least one parent. In the future I'm sure we will see changes that enable working parents to have enough flexibility to meet the demands of their work without compromising the emotional health of their children — or without neglecting the relationships between one another. Flexible working hours, job sharing, family travel together on business trips, and the mandatory permission by employers to allow parents to attend school conferences and special events in which their children participate will be among the changes to take place. If, as a society, we consider the family an important unit, we must make changes in the practices of institutions to support and enhance the family.

I'm very impressed by the fact that young people today are looking for close ties with one other person. There seems to be a resurgence of the desire to share, to want physical closeness, and to be open and honest about their expectations of one another. Nothing could enhance our society more than having people who want to live together, love each other, and enjoy sharing. Many of the conflicts that today lead to divorce will in the future be talked out before marriage. I'm convinced that, more and more, people will approach their relationships and commitments in a way that's going to be considerably more honest than it has been in the past.

You will notice as you read my responses to the problems people have put before me that my recommendations are not in recipe form. I have attempted to provide knowledge and insight into the *meaning* of problems and then have explained the consequences of the various actions you might take in handling the problem.

Ask Dr. Salk

Teaching Manners
to a Toddler

When should you start to teach a toddler manners? Our three-year-old sits at the dinner table with us, and my husband's constantly telling her to eat with her spoon and fork properly, to sit still at the table, and to say "please" and "thank you" for everything. I think she's too young for all this instruction, but my husband says it's never too early to learn good manners. When is a small child capable of learning about manners? And are they that important for little children to know?

I think your child is old enough to learn table manners, but they should be taught in an atmosphere of warmth, under-standing, and patience. If you are severe and demanding about her actions at the table, and punitive when she fails to behave properly, she will come to dread mealtime.

When children are around eighteen months of age, they begin to imitate the things their parents do. In this way they will pick up your bad habits as well as your good ones. If you are careless in your mealtime habits, and reach and grab, your daughter will probably do the same; but if you set a good example, she should follow suit.

By respecting her wishes to imitate you, you can encourage good manners with smiles, a continued recognition of her efforts, and a positive attitude. Prepare yourself for her awkwardness, mistakes, and a certain amount of spilling and dropping. It may be hard for her to maneuver utensils and plates gracefully at this age, but this is precisely where your responsibility comes in. You have to guide her patiently and give

1

her the opportunity of doing things for herself while tolerating some of her errors. If she doesn't make mistakes, she will never be able to learn.

I find that making a game out of everything is sometimes the best way to get across important information. In the mind of a young child there's a bit of magic in finding that when you pass the salt to a grownup, he or she automatically says "thank you" with a smile. Exaggeration from time to time is also a good way to get your point across; if you are overly emphatic in your politeness, a little child is sure to notice that what you are doing must be very important indeed. On occasion, if you find your own manners flagging, your child would probably be amused if you were to say, "Oops! You had better take the salt back from me again — I forgot to say thank you!"

Children who are well mannered and respectful of other people's feelings generally have more freedom to accompany their parents on visits; they are usually completely welcomed by grownups, who find it a delight to be with children with these qualities. While it is possible to get good manners across by hammering and nagging at children in a harsh and punitive way, the same goals can be accomplished in an atmosphere of pleasantness. When this occurs, these values become part of the children's normal behavior on the basis of desire rather than on the basis of fear.

❦

The Importance of Toys

Our four-year-old constantly loses or breaks his toys, and I wonder if there's any point in my trying to correct this situation. After all, are toys really that important?

Play is an essential part of the learning experience of young children, and it is important to provide toys that are stimulating and help develop skills that can be applied to everyday life. Such toys are tools that should be treated properly, and it's important for children to learn to take care of their possessions and be aware of their responsibilities in keeping track of them.

In some instances, your child may break or lose his toys because they are so unstimulating or poorly made that he simply loses interest in them. Do your best to provide him with constructive and sturdy playthings, and indicate to him by word and example the care with which they should be treated. This should go a long way toward teaching him this important developmental lesson.

❦

Tasting Liquor From a Parent's Drink

At weddings and special occasions, my husband allows our children — they're eight and ten — to sip from his glass of champagne, wine, or beer. More and more now, the children tease to have a drink, while the adults smile as though they're amused by the whole thing. I think this is turning into a bad habit, but my husband laughs and says it's nothing at all to worry about. What do you think?

When you take a strongly prohibitive view on something like alcohol, you tend to make liquor seem enticing and a drink of it adventurous. On the other hand, viewing its consumption as something cute and charming can make it equally enticing but for a different reason — a child then sees it as a means for gaining parental recognition by doing "adorable" things. In either case, you can increase a child's motivation to drink these "forbidden" liquids.

The moment you offer attention, either negative or positive, you are giving alcohol a value that goes beyond a matter of simple curiosity about its taste. If this happens, you can intensify your children's desire for alcohol. They may later use alcohol as a way of defying you, hurting you when they are angry, or use it as a vehicle for showing their independence or even their attractiveness.

I think the situation calls for some concern on your part, but I wouldn't take the position that these little sips will inevitably lead to alcoholism. A casual attitude is the best one. I see nothing wrong with letting children of this age sip champagne, wine, or beer out of curiosity. And if you handle the matter nonchalantly and show no undue concern or evidence of being charmed, in all likelihood the desire for further drinks will diminish.

❦

Conceived Before Marriage — What to Tell a Child

Our daughter is now twelve but was conceived about four months before my husband and I were actually married. We've never made a point of concealing her real birthdate or the date of our anniversary — our marriage has been a happy one, and we celebrate it regularly — but now we realize that it's only a matter of time before our daughter puts these facts together and figures out what happened. Should we be the ones to talk to her about it, or should we wait to see if she ever mentions the sub-

4

ject? Is such upsetting news going to affect the nice feelings between our daughter and ourselves?

As always, I believe in being honest with children. They are far more capable of dealing with the truth than many grown-ups believe. If you have a good relationship with your daughter, there is no way it can be damaged by her finding out that she was conceived before your marriage. The love that exists in your home transcends any possible damage that could come about by her knowing the truth. In fact, you run far more risk of damaging your credibility and the bond of trust between you by hiding the facts or distorting them. Let her know how much you and your husband loved each other and how that love led to her birth. Explain that the actual date of a marriage has no bearing at all on those feelings of concern and affection.

There was a time in the past when it might have been embarrassing for a child to learn that she was conceived out of wedlock. Fortunately, we are living at a time when there is greater acceptance of such all-too-human circumstances. This news that you consider upsetting is likely to be received in a matter-of-fact way by most people today.

❦

Teaching the Value of Money

My children have reached the ages of five and seven, and I'm wondering what to do about giving them money. At what age should children start receiving allowances, and what should parents tell their children about the value of money and how it is to be used?

There is no specific age that I can recommend for starting a child on an allowance because many other factors are involved. In order to make an allowance meaningful for a child, he or she should understand what money is used for, that to have it one must earn it, and that once spent it cannot easily be retrieved.

Children often have unrealistic notions of where money comes from and how to get more. Some children think that you simply go to the bank and money is given to you. Others think that real money isn't necessary at all, that a plastic card enables you to get whatever you want.

Ideally, children should be taught that work, effort, and honest ingenuity enable people to obtain money. Whatever the source of your money, explain to your child how you and your family earn it. Make your explanation as concrete and simple as you can. Then point out that as part of a family unit, each member of the family benefits from the money that comes into your household. Although everyone in the family doesn't work to earn that money directly, everyone must share in the variety of jobs involved in maintaining the household. By doing so, everyone in the family is entitled to some share of the money that is earned. By getting across the idea that everyone is entitled to some of the money that comes in, but that each person also has to contribute some of the work, you reinforce the importance of family unity and shared responsibility.

When you offer your children an allowance, let them know that it is theirs to spend or save, but that you will offer some advice about how to use it in a satisfying yet careful manner. Explain that grownups frequently go to other people for advice on what to do with their money. While it's necessary to emphasize the importance of money, it's equally necessary not to place so much value on it that your children feel they have to hoard it and become unwilling to spend anything.

❦

Your Child's Allowance

My eight-year-old son came in the door the other day with a sleazy-looking and overpriced Super-Hero Spaceship that he had purchased with his allowance. When I told him to return it, a great scene ensued because he said it was "his money." Should children be allowed to do whatever they want with their allowances? Should I just keep my mouth shut when my kids come home with something they've bought that seems ridiculous to me? And after they've wasted their money on a piece of junk, should I allow them to wheedle me into giving them an "advance" on their allowance because they've run out of money that week?

In principle, children should be allowed to do whatever they want with their allowance, providing they don't do anything that is destructive to themselves or anyone else. On the other hand, it's important for parents to provide guidance to children in learning how to spend their money. While you cannot absolutely dictate what they should do with their money, don't hesitate to offer your opinions or reactions to what they buy — as long as you do so in a manner that is constructive and not deprecatory. Ridiculing a child, or telling him that he's stupid, doesn't do any good. Explaining to him that what he has bought is a poor value for his money, and telling him why, would be far more useful.

In order for a child to learn how to postpone immediate gratification for greater satisfaction in the long run — a very important lesson to be learned in life — you should avoid bailing him out and giving him an advance on his allowance. This is certainly the case if your child tends to use poor judgment and buys things impulsively. However, if on occasion your child has used sound judgment in managing financial matters but needs more money during a given week, I see no harm in your advancing some money to him. Understandably, this gives you certain options and puts you in a position to judge how he spends his money, but that is precisely what guidance is. It provides you with a chance to encourage good spending habits in your child while discouraging extravagance.

❦

Child Supervision For Working Parents

My husband and I both work. Until now, we've had someone in the house until just before we return home. But now that my son is fourteen and my daughter is ten, I am wondering if it is necessary to have an adult present after school. Can children of this age supervise themselves?

Many children of this age can supervise themselves, but having an adult present at home after school should not necessarily be for supervision. Perhaps more important than supervision is the feeling that there is someone at home who cares, who can give recognition, and who is available to handle any problems that might arise. Many children who come home to an empty house feel resentful, and sometimes feel sufficiently angry to be destructive. Other children, similar in age, seem capable of handling responsibility and can even do family chores after school, which gives them a sense of pride and an opportunity for parental recognition for making things easier for the whole family. When parents show pride and appreciation for this kind of help, there is usually little or no need to pressure children for further help.

I suggest that you discuss the question of having an adult present after school with both your children. Be responsive to their wishes and let them help you make the decision. Let them know that you recognize that they are growing up and perhaps they themselves feel there's little need to have someone taking care of them for the few hours between the end of school and your returning from work. Don't pressure them or leave them with the idea that if they choose to continue having someone present at home that it's a sign of immaturity or irresponsibility. Let them know you understand that it might feel more comfortable to have someone to talk to and be with until you get home.

As a general rule, I think parents should be open with their children in discussing issues like these. Children enjoy participating in decision making particularly when it comes to family issues since it gives them a greater sense of importance in the family and helps enhance a strong sense of self-worth. When parents engage children in family decisions, it also provides a good model for how families should function. Shared responsibility, shared decision making, respect for individuality, and compassion are important human elements that come into play when issues arise and are resolved in this way.

❦

The Effects of Baby Talk

My husband's parents talk baby talk to our four-year-old, and now my husband has started doing it, too. Aren't all these cutesy words for everything from food ("nummies") to blanket ("blankey") harmful to a small child's language development?

While the words themselves won't ultimately prove harmful to your child's language development, they can affect his or her self-image and social relationships. A four-year-old child who attends nursery school and has a vocabulary filled with "cutesy words" may be teased by other children or regarded as immature by his teachers. Also, if your four-year-old visits a friend's house and politely asks for "nummies," confusion is likely to result, and the child's attempts at meaningful communication will be impeded.

A child of four is perfectly capable of understanding words that are used correctly. When adults cling to baby talk even when children grow older, it tends to keep the children infantile by keeping them from using appropriately mature language. This sort of thing is more reflective of the adult's need than it is of the child's; some people enjoy keeping young children dependent and babylike, even when the child is capable of and struggles for more independence. No wonder that many children resent being talked down to in this way. Children are far more trusting and respectful of people who speak to them in a forthright manner that does not demean them.

I used to find it hilariously funny to listen to my daughter Pia's imitations of adults who spoke baby talk to her. Whenever anyone would launch into a high-pitched, elaborately enunciated monologue loaded with baby talk in an attempt to engage Pia in conversation, her reaction was always incredulous: "Why does that lady talk like such a baby?" she would say. "Why can't she talk like a grownup?"

❦

When and How to Explain Reproduction and Sex

My child is three years old and is already beginning to ask about where he "came from." When should parents begin to discuss sex with their children? And can you give some guidelines about what children really want to know at what age, and just how much information is appropriate to give them?

Parents should begin discussions of sex with young children as soon as the children begin to ask questions. Children are by nature very curious and inquisitive, and parents should nurture and satisfy this curiosity by giving them the information they want. This not only motivates toward further learning but provides them with the knowledge they need to grow and deal with life's situations and problems.

In order to be able to deal with their children's sexual curiosity, it's important for parents themselves to be informed. Admittedly, many adults are not as knowledgeable about sexual matters as they should be, and many have received misinformation during their own early years. If this is the case, parents should make a point of educating themselves, perhaps by talking to other adults in community or church groups, consulting books (maybe even ones intended for their children!), or doctors or therapists about the correct advice to give to their children.

Parents who are unsure of their own knowledge or information tend to turn the responsibility over to someone else — the family doctor, a teacher, a member of the clergy, or even a more "relaxed" relative or family friend. In my opinion, this is very unwise because it makes a child wonder why his or her own parents don't answer these questions themselves. I believe that outside "professionals" or authority figures are no more qualified than the parents themselves. In fact, I think they're *less* qualified simply because they have less understanding of a particular child's view of the world. Also, parents are far more sensitive to what their children want to know and to the words that can best be used to get this information across. But most important, even though school and community programs can be helpful later in supplying additional information, sex education should begin in a child's own family.

The first questions most children ask are about the reproductive process and not about deeper sexual emotions. The age at which children begin to ask questions varies. It can start as early as two years of age, but in my experience, it peaks between the ages of three and four. This, of course, depends upon many circumstances. The arrival of a new baby brother or sister might trigger questions; so might the birth of a litter of kittens. Often a child begins by asking questions about sex by wondering about how families get started or "how grandma got to be *your* mother." Other children simply ask, "Where do babies come from?" or, "How did I get here?" When these questions arise, parents should answer honestly, using correct terminology to explain things on a level a child can understand. While some parents feel the explanation should be in the context of "the birds and the bees," I believe this can be irrelevant or confusing to a child. Children sense a parent's reluctance to give information straightforwardly and can easily interpret an oblique approach to their questions as an indication that these are forbidden topics. And never tell a child, "You're too young to know about these things." This answer will not make the question go away; it will only make a child turn elsewhere for answers and will indicate to children that you have no respect for their curiosity.

A child should be told that a baby starts to grow when a sperm from inside a man's body comes together with a very tiny egg (no bigger than the size of a pinhead) inside a woman's body. Explain that it takes nine months for that tiny egg to grow into a full-size baby and that the baby grows inside the woman's body in a place called the uterus. (Don't, for goodness sake, say "stomach," but explain just where the uterus is, "below or near the stomach.") The baby's food comes from the food the woman eats, and the baby gets everything else it needs from inside the woman's body. Let the child know that as the baby gets larger and larger, the woman's body gets bigger and bigger in the place where the baby is growing, and that when the baby is ready to be born, the woman usually goes to the hospital and has the help of a doctor or nurse or midwife to help the baby be born.

A child will probably ask, "How does the baby get out?" This should be explained by saying, "Most babies are born through the vagina. The vagina gets bigger when the baby is ready to be born, and then it gets smaller again after the baby has come out." It's not necessary to go into detail about caesarian section unless the child asks specifically about it or unless it's personally relevant to that child. If, for example, one of your children was born by caesarian section, you may want to explain it in more detail.

The question parents find most difficult, and one that a child is almost sure to ask, is, "How does the sperm from a man get inside the woman's body?" You need not wait for a child to ask about this — in fact, it might be best to show a willingness to offer this information. Ask the child, "Wouldn't you like to know how it happens?" If a child seems interested, your explanation might be something like this: "When a man and a woman love each other a lot, they enjoy hugging each other and kissing each other. This gives them very warm and loving feelings, which sometimes makes both the man and woman want to have the man put his penis in the woman's vagina. This usually makes them both feel very good, and often sperm comes through the man's penis and out into where the egg is in the woman's body. When one tiny sperm becomes connected to the tiny egg, the baby starts to grow."

It's always helpful for parents to have a book available with illustrations of what the egg, sperm, and growing baby look like in a woman's uterus. One of my favorite books for this purpose is *Did the Sun Shine Before You Were Born?* written by Sol and Judith Gordon and published by the Third Press. These books can also be helpful for adults — who may learn things that *they* did not know.

❦

Watching Painful Topics on TV

My eight- and ten-year-olds started to watch "Holocaust" when it was on television, and I turned it off thinking they would be terribly upset by it. But my sister-in-law feels that children must know that such things as the Holocaust have occurred, that they should see newsreel footage of the boat people and starving children in Cambodia so that they will become aware and compassionate. Is she right? Should children watch programs dealing with painful topics and the sufferings of others?

In general, programs that deal with human suffering serve to sensitize children toward the situations of others and make them aware of important historical events. Such programs help children realistically understand the ravages of war and the grave injustice and cruelty that can occur in the world. The resulting upset, outrage, and horror that such programs can cause are entirely appropriate.

When you allow your children to view television programs and news documentaries of this nature, however, you should be on hand to help them deal with the feelings they arouse. Watch with them, and openly express your own horror that such terrible things can happen. If you sit by passively, viewing such programs without expressing sensitivity or outrage, your children may feel that you yourself don't care when human beings are demeaned and tortured and destroyed. You must make it clear that you are moved and deeply concerned about what you see and that everyone must do what he or she can to prevent these injustices in the lives of all people.

It is also true that not all children should be encouraged to view such programs. Some children are unusually sensitive, some have emotional problems, and others with extreme fears may become very upset and disorganized by these programs. It is up to parents to decide how much each child is able to handle.

Television Violence

Even on the cartoons my kids watch on Saturday mornings, the characters sometimes slug and batter each other — and on other shows they watch, crooks and good guys battle it out, and there's shooting and bloodshed. I know people have been upset about violence on TV for a long time now, but are there indications that children are really affected by it? What are your feelings about kids watching violence on TV? And should I make an effort to curtail their watching these programs?

I certainly believe that children should be discouraged from watching violence on television and should instead be encouraged to view programs of an informational or educational nature. Personally, I would like to see violence on television eliminated altogether. There are indications that children who view a great deal of it are indeed affected by it. However, it is fair to add that children are exposed to violence elsewhere as well, in fairy tales and stories, including many of the biblical ones, and that it is realistic to acknowledge that children must learn to deal with hostility and aggressiveness. Excessive violence, however, can only serve to densensitize children and make them think that such behavior is permissible.

In general, children past the age of five know that the slugging and battering that take place in some Saturday morning cartoons or adventure shows is extremely exaggerated and at times totally unrealistic. Children under the age of five, however, may see characters such as the Three Stooges knocking one another about with no apparent harm and may expect the same carefree consequences to result in real life and to imitate what they see. Actions in cartoons or "comedies" are viewed by young children in a very literal and concrete way, and we've all heard of tragedies that sometimes occur when little children attempt to fly "like Superman" from a real height. Children need help in learning to differentiate between fantasy and reality. Adults must recognize these possible consequences and try to prevent them from occurring by monitoring what children see and anticipating their responses seriously. Otherwise, children will be vulnerable to grave dangers.

🍎

Television as "Baby-Sitter"

I hear people making derisive remarks about "using the television set as a baby-sitter." But I admit to it! Sometimes I'm so tired or have so much to do that I'm happy to have my kids — they're three and five and nine) — transfixed in front of the TV set. Am I doing a terrible thing by allowing this to happen?

No, you're not, as long as this does not happen frequently, and you are aware of what it is your children are watching. But parents should not allow indiscriminate television watching to become an "addiction" — one that children can come to feel is "endorsed" by their parents. Then, later on, when parents attempt to cut down viewing time, there is great exasperation on everyone's part. That is why rules limiting the time and the kind of programs children are allowed to watch should be established from the first.

Unquestionably, children should have other forms of stimulation, and parents should do everything they can to help them engage in a wider range of activities. Reading, musical and sports activities, and creative play with paints and toys are only some of the possibilities. Television watching should be only one possibility among many others.

🍎

Being "Hooked" on TV Soap Operas

My husband makes fun of the soap operas I watch regularly — he teases me because he says my brain is going to "turn to mush." But I find myself really caught up in them. I turn on my set as I'm doing household chores, and they make me feel better, for reasons I can't quite explain. Is soap-opera watching a harmful waste of time?

I believe that soap operas have positive virtues and do not deserve the ridicule that some people give them. They are often based on problems and situations that occur in real life, and in many cases the plots and the interactions among the characters provide real insight into human nature. Some people feel better from watching soap operas if for no other reason than they see that the problems they face in everyday life are similar to those that other people have. And in any event, the drama of human emotions dealt with on daytime television can be much deeper and more meaningful than many of the fast-paced comedy and adventure shows that often characterize evening television.

As far as your brain "turning to mush," it won't do so from watching soap operas any more than it might from doing tedious, repetitive household chores. The only problem that might occur is if your habit of watching prevents you from getting through your day without adequately coping with your life and your family. Any activity that is carried to such an extreme has a compulsive quality to it, and you should examine the feelings that may be behind your escape into television watching.

❦

Teenagers and the Orthodontist

*The dentist peered into our thirteen-year-old's mouth and an-
nounced she should have braces. It's true — her teeth are
crooked. But the thought of braces upsets her terribly, and she
refuses to have "all that metal stuff" in her mouth that will
"hurt and make her look ugly." Should we insist that she go
through with a procedure that the dentist says could take two
or three years? I'm sure that when she gets older, she'll thank
us for her straight, beautiful teeth — but is all this agony and
carrying on in the interim worth it?*

You may not have as much agony as you anticipate if you go
through with the procedure. Remember, a thirteen-year-old is
inclined to reject anything that her parents suggest. In a very
histrionic way, your daughter is attempting to assert herself
and, at the same time, is very vain. Perhaps you should openly
agree with her that braces are not pretty and that they certainly
do create some discomfort, but that the long-range benefits
would be to *her* advantage and not yours. Ask her to discuss it
with friends who already have braces; her peer group may
come up with more effective arguments than you might even
think of.

Another approach is to call a cooling-off period. Tell your
daughter that "I'm not going to insist on your doing this, even
though I know someday you'll appreciate it. It's your mouth
and your appearance, and if you want to let things go on this
way, you may. But I think you ought to consider it, and when
we go back to the dentist again in a few weeks, you can let him
know your decision after you have given it more thought." In
this way you will be showing consideration for her feelings, giving her the independence to make her own choice, and allowing
her to restructure her view of the situation at a later date.

I must admit that I was faced with a problem the opposite of
yours. When my daughter, Pia, was eight and a half, she

18

thought that teenagers who had braces were "cute." When she visited her dentist she kept asking, "When will you put braces in my mouth?" When he told her, "You may not need braces," my daughter seemed terribly disappointed. Her desire for braces was so intense that on occasion I found her bending paper clips into the form of braces and putting them in her mouth, which she then smilingly admired in the mirror. Children are not only the greatest joy in the world, but they are sometimes the greatest mystery!

❦

Character Evaluation by the School

My child came home from the fourth grade yesterday with her "character evaluation" report. The teacher had "rated" each child, on an official school form, as to his or her qualities of "leadership," "cooperation," "potential for achievement," and so forth. I was very distressed by this. I think it's wrong for teachers to make such "evaluations." Can you see any purpose for children being rated in such a way by a subjective observer? And isn't such a thing likely to give children an image of themselves that may not be productive for them later in life?

Yes, it could. But what is most distressing about this is the immediate discomfort it creates for the child, as well as the questionable criteria for making these evaluations in the first place. The teacher certainly places himself or herself in a position of great power in making such judgments, and I can see no way in which such a report given in this manner can have beneficial effects. If there are weaknesses in a child's personality, this sort of evaluation can undermine the child's self-confidence even more.

19

Children take reports like this very seriously, and the fact that they are so subjective and are made by someone who sees the child under limited circumstances and from his or her own particular point of view makes the "evaluation" potentially dangerous or, at best, very distressing. If there is genuine concern on the part of school staff over a child's character development, a teacher should speak in private with the child in the presence of the parents. In this way, a teacher could *communicate* his or her *impressions* of a child's behavior, and the issue could then be discussed in a manner that might lead to improved behavior on the part of the child. But when a teacher simply presents a written evaluation, there is virtually no opportunity for any input or feedback by others so crucially involved. I think it is entirely appropriate for you and other parents to arrange a meeting with the teachers involved to discuss this matter.

❦

Bragging and Exaggerating

My eight-year-old is always quoting "facts" that his friend has told him — that the bionic man is his uncle (he isn't), that his father used to play for the Oakland Raiders (he didn't), and so on — stories that my son believes and quotes endlessly to us as the gospel truth. How can we tell our son that his friend isn't really the authority our boy thinks he is, without making our son feel foolish?

It is very common for children to exaggerate details of their lives, even to the point of constructing "facts" that are a mixture of lies and fantasy. Children use this sort of sensationalism to fascinate their friends and at the same time gain a sense of importance in the eyes of their peers. In fact, children not only act out make-believe situations in play but may also even come to believe what they have conjured up in their own minds.

Explain to your son that even though it is very natural and loyal of him to take his friend at his word, the friend is making up these stories about his uncle and father simply to impress others. An eight-year-old is capable of understanding that sometimes children feel a little weak inside and that they tell such stories to make themselves seem more important. Your reaction will help give your son some understanding of his friend's motivation and at the same time should protect him from feeling foolish about believing these "facts."

❦

Helping a Child Accept Defeat

Our thirteen-year-old spent weeks building a go-cart for a race to be held during a local fair. To the dismay of all of us, he finished nearly last in the race. Since his defeat over a week ago, he has sulked silently and the go-cart has sat idle in the garage. We've tried telling him, "It's not whether you win or lose . . ." But that just makes him angry. What else can a parent say to console a disheartened child? Is his reaction normal?

This is *not* an abnormal reaction. Your child is simply and naturally disappointed in losing. In all likelihood, he had many fantasies during the weeks he built his go-cart. At one time or other during his labors, he must have imagined the applause as he reached the finish line first and received a gold trophy while his proud parents stood by. In addition to this discrepancy between fantasy and reality, he also surely feels the frustration of hard work that did not result in the rewards he hoped for.

When children are disheartened in this way, it's best to show compassion and allow them to experience these feelings for an appropriate amount of time, rather than attempt to convince them that they "shouldn't take it so hard." Tell your son, "I know you are very disappointed because you did such a good job and still came in nearly last." When you show understanding for your son's feelings, he is apt to verbalize more of his own thoughts and should be willing to discuss with you constructive ideas about what made the other carts so much faster or what driving techniques were used. He then may be willing to work again to increase his chances of success for the next race. You also can remind him, as you talk, of other areas in which he does excel.

While it is often hard for a child to accept failure when he or she has worked so hard to achieve success, facing this harsh reality is one of life's lessons. While parental comfort and acceptance can do much to temper a child's frustration, you also must accept the fact that it will simply take time for your son to get over his disappointment.

❦

Choosing to Be Single and Have a Child

I'm a woman in my early thirties, with a good job and a lovely apartment — and no particular inclination to get married. But lately I've thought more and more about having a baby, husband or not. I feel I could provide a loving, stable home for a child. What are your thoughts about unwed mothers? In today's society, is there any real reason a single woman shouldn't raise a child alone?

I do think it is *possible* for a single woman to raise a child successfully. Many widows and divorced women have done so. But, for them, the undertaking was a matter of necessity rather than choice; and for most of them, there must have been many hardships. I don't encourage a single woman to raise a baby alone. It is easy to fantasize about rearing a lovely, happy baby that fits into an already well-organized life. But while the fantasy is appealing, the reality may be something quite different. The commitment involved in parenthood is enormous and requires many changes in a person's lifestyle. Raising a child involves not only pleasures and satisfactions but also very real financial and emotional burdens, as well as uncertainties and anxieties about the future. Your good job, your lovely apartment, and the personal freedom you now enjoy will all be affected by the needs and demands of a new baby. I don't mean to make parenthood sound unpleasant, I simply want to impress every potential parent — married or single — with its responsibilities.

If you as a single person honestly feel that you can provide a loving, stable home for a child, consider making the children of friends and relatives a part of your life. Invite them for afternoon adventures or weekend visits. Children love to go on trips with friendly grownups, and you might consider spending part of your vacation with a friend's child. You might also consider volunteer work with children in your community. In this way you can share in the joys and satisfactions of having children without taking on the sole responsibility for the full-time and long-range care of a child.

My deepest concern is for the welfare of children. And in my mind it would be unfair to a child to be born into a one-parent situation where the baby's needs would be compromised from the very start.

❦

Having an Only Child

Our son is a year old, and we have decided for several good reasons that he will be our only child. However, we are often told by friends and family that a child "needs brothers and sisters" so he can learn to "share." We don't want our little boy to be a spoiled only child. Is there danger of that?

There is no reason at all why you can't bring up an only child to be well adjusted, well liked, and respectful of other people's feelings, and I admire you for making the decision to have only one child if this is truly what you want. In fact, your son is likely to get a good deal of individual time and attention, which is so essential to the emotional health of children during their early years. And don't let anyone give you the argument that you will be depriving your only child of a friend. For every only child I have known who wished for a brother or sister, there have been at least a dozen others who later had siblings and viewed them with both hostility and jealousy.

As far as "sharing" is concerned, when your child is three years of age he can attend a nursery school, which will give him an opportunity for companionship with other children. In a setting such as this, he will learn to deal with the frustrations that arise when he wants something that another child has. True, when children interact with one another, they develop internal controls and a tolerance for frustration that helps them become more socialized and capable of dealing with freedom — but these learning experiences are clearly not limited to families with brothers and sisters.

Some "only" children do seem obnoxious. In my experience it's because their parents tended to overindulge them out of guilt and give them *things* instead of time and attention. Some parents avoid frustrating their children at any cost, supposedly to prevent psychological trauma. These children rarely learn to deal with frustration and frequently develop the feeling that the world revolves around them. But this can happen to any child, regardless of whether he or she is an "only" child.

❣

Mixed Feelings About Parenthood

My husband and I have talked about having a family — and although he says he'll go along with it if that's what I want, the fact is that he's never been especially interested in other people's children. I wonder if this is a warning signal that we shouldn't have children of our own? Does his current indifference indicate he wouldn't be a good father?

Many men seem somewhat lukewarm in their attitude toward children in general, but after having children of their own, they revel in their parental involvement. While this change can happen, however, it is by no means always the case. There is an even better chance that your husband's indifferent attitude will *not* turn to great enthusiasm.

Raising children is a tremendous commitment that takes a great deal of time, effort, and patience. It's a responsibility that is more easily shared by two people than carried by one. If you do decide to have children, prepare yourself for the fact that you may have to assume the primary burden of raising them, and it will change your life in ways you never could have expected. While the joys and pleasures are enormous, the frustrations and problems will sometimes seem overwhelming.

I see nothing wrong with people choosing not to have children if they lack the enthusiasm for the undertaking or feel that it will change their lifestyle too drastically. I suggest you examine your own motives for wanting children and give very careful thought to the possibility that your husband's current indifference will continue even with children of his own. If you are prepared as realistically as possible for what might happen, you will be in a better position to make a decision and then deal with all the possibilities that might arise because of it.

❧

Playing with Guns

My son, who will soon be three, has developed a great fascination with guns. He says that all he wants for his birthday is guns; at play he will use a finger or stick for a gun and gets great pleasure from "shooting" airplanes that fly by, or just about anything else for that matter. My husband feels we should go ahead and let him have a toy gun, and then when the newness wears off, he'll forget about it and go on to something else. But I feel this would encourage him, and he would think we approve of what he is doing. Is our son's behavior normal, and how should we handle it?

This is a very common play situation that many young children engage in — and it often causes chagrin for parents who are strong advocates of nonviolence. Most children, however, spontaneously pass out of this "shoot-em-up" stage and become equally fascinated with other things as they get older and their range of interests increases.

Nevertheless, during this time it's important for you to convey your values about violence in general and guns in particular. Making an issue of confiscating a toy gun is useless, however; a child will use fingers or a stick for an imaginary gun, and your prohibitive attitude will only make the activity more alluring. On the other hand, participating in the ritual by actually buying a toy weapon, or standing by indifferently while it is fired, would indeed encourage him and make it seem that you approve.

I suggest that you make it very clear that you don't like to see your son playing in this manner. Let him know that guns can hurt people badly, sometimes even kill them, and that you would much prefer to see him have fun in other kinds of ways. By making your feelings and displeasure known — without over-reacting to such an extent that the forbidden gunplay becomes even more desirable — you should get your message across. And, in time, this should cease to be a problem.

❦

The Serious Teenager's Drive for Excellence

My thirteen-year-old son takes everything so seriously. It's necessary for him to excel in whatever he does, from schoolwork to athletic games — and if he fails to make the highest grades or win the top honors, he becomes very frustrated and upset and takes no joy in what he has accomplished. We're of course proud of him — but worried, too. Why is he trying so hard to prove himself?

In a sense, your son is carrying to an extreme a situation that most parents would find desirable: He is taking work and responsibilities seriously and is highly motivated to achieve. He must sense your approval of his seriousness and hard work; the problem is that he approaches these things compulsively and has simply gone too far in trying to prove himself.

I believe your son unconsciously associates achievement with the winning of parental love and approval. His intense behavior and frustration over imperfection results from an idea deep inside himself that anything short of "excellence" is equivalent to the loss of your esteem and support.

It is hard for mothers and fathers to encourage children to take all their responsibilities seriously and praise them for their accomplishments and yet not have it relate in some way in the child's mind with parental approval and acceptance. You must reassure your son in whatever ways you can that, although you are indeed proud of him, your love is not dependent on his "performance" in school or athletic activities. Make it clear that your basic affection for him is unaffected by external prizes or awards. It sounds, however, as if his compulsive desire to excel and his fear of rejection are so deeply rooted that you may be unable to get this message through to him. I believe it will take competent professional psychological help to enable your son to understand his compulsions — and to make peace with himself in a way that allows him to enjoy his work and his success without equating it so closely with your love.

❦

Child Care for Working Parents

I'll be going back to work soon, and my child is almost three. What kind of child-care situation do you recommend for children whose parents must work, and why?

When children are under three years of age, they generally need a great deal of individual adult attention. In general, they're not ready for organized play with other children on a sustained basis. More often than not, they tend to play by themselves, alongside other children, and frequently grab what they want when they want it. Until three, many children tend to be negativistic and openly defiant. Since they also imitate the behavior of people around them, they frequently become more aggressive and show more destructive behavior if they've been in close contact for long periods of time with other children in the range of two years of age. I don't mean to imply that on a child's third birthday he magically turns into a cooperative and trusting human being! It doesn't happen that abruptly, but, in general, three-year-olds show much more cooperative behavior and can benefit psychologically from being in an organized play situation such as a nursery school. In fact, it can serve as a very positive experience for a child and help him learn to deal with peer situations.

It would be wonderful if nursery schools or preschools could be in proximity with the parents' work place. This would enable parents to spend their lunch time with their children. Not only would this give them an opportunity for close contact with one another but it also would serve to give the child the feeling that his parents are prominent in his life. When children spend little time with their parents, no matter how good the quality of the time, the parents' importance in the child's life is substantially diminished.

Notice, I've not used the words "day-care center" but have talked of nursery school. The term "day care" places emphasis on the parents' need to have their day taken care of, while the term "school" or "child-care facility" focuses more on the needs of the child. This is not simply a semantic issue but one, I think, that reflects the growing tendency in our society to ignore the needs of our children and focus on the needs of adults. Understandably, many parents must work and therefore require help for the care of their children. I am a strong advocate of the best in child care. Since children at this age require a great deal of one-to-one contact, I would like to look toward better solutions for the child-care problem than compromise by placing little children in day-care facilities that are not geared to meet the psychological and emotional needs of children at that age.

❧

Back to Work After Childbirth

I'll be going back to work shortly after the birth of my child. What actual effects will this have? What should I do to make up for my absence? Do children whose parents aren't with them every moment of the day need special reassurances or care?

I don't believe that parents need to be with their children every moment of the day, but children clearly need to feel the presence and responsiveness of their parents for prolonged periods of time in the course of each day, particularly when they are very young. They need consistency, and they need to feel that they are important in the lives of their parents. If your child spends most of her waking hours with someone other than you, she will understandably grow more attached to that person and be more responsive to that person's patterns of behavior than yours. If at all possible, I urge you to spend a few hours in the middle of each day with your baby. (Ideally, I'd like to see parents of very young children have flexible working hours that enable one parent or the other to do this.) If you are gone for perhaps three to four hours at a time and return for an hour or two in between, your importance in the life of your child will be substantially greater than it would be if you are gone for eight to nine hours a day at a stretch. If it's not possible for you to return home, perhaps you can have whoever is caring for your child bring her to where you work. This would enable you to be with your child and feed your child during that period of time. Many mothers I've spoken with who have been unable or have chosen not to spend considerable amounts of time with their children in the early years feel guilty about having neglected their children. They also feel as if they've been deprived of an important aspect of their own lives by not having been with their children during those very important early days.

I'm hard put to justify turning little children over to other people to raise because the effects of these early disruptions in a child's relationship with parents have such damaging effects later on. In our society we spend enormous sums of money trying to repair the damages caused by disrupted parent-child relationships in these early formative years. It would be far easier to prevent the damage by modifying our approach to children to preserve the integrity of the parent-child bond while still enabling parents to carry out their work responsibilities.

❦

Working Couples and the Question of Parenthood

My husband and I, who are in our early thirties, are talking about the possibility of having a child, but I am worried about whether I could be a good parent and at the same time continue to work in an office where I have a considerable amount of responsibility. Do you think that with a good five-day-week sitter-housekeeper, my retired father-in-law on tap for emergencies, and a great deal of attention from both parents evenings and weekends, we could provide the proper climate for raising a child? Or do you think that the stress of holding a full-time job might be too great for me and thus too stressful for an infant or young child? My husband and I both feel we want one child, but I also would like to continue in my profession, where I have worked very hard to establish myself.

It's easy to have a child, but it's hard to be a parent. Parenthood is the most important job a human being can take on in life and therefore requires that adult couples give very serious consideration to whether or not they can meet the needs of a child before undertaking this monumental task. In my mind, it is highly unfair to bring a child into this world and turn him over to someone else to raise. All children deserve the right to be wanted. I can understand that you and your husband would like an infant, but I question whether you should become parents in view of the fact that you seem so heavily committed to other things. I admire people who can be sufficiently honest with themselves to make the decision that they will *not* have a child because they cannot give it the time and attention it requires. Life involves many compromises and many sacrifices. If your life leaves little room for being able to provide the best conditions for raising a child, then I think you should consider bypassing parenthood. Perhaps you can satisfy your parental needs by having the children of friends or relatives spend time with you on weekends or even holidays. Many parents would find it a welcome relief to have their children spend time with relatives and friends, and in many ways this would give you all the advantages of parenthood without the disadvantages.

The Depressed, Unemployed Young College Graduate

Our son graduated from college and spent all summer looking for a job — without success. He now seems to have given up, and spends his time either hanging around the house or drifting around aimlessly with his unemployed friends. He seems depressed, and we just don't know what to do to snap him out of it. Is it natural for a young man to be as down in the dumps and unmotivated as this?

It is natural for any person to feel depressed and discouraged after a long period of unsuccessful job hunting. It's even more understandable when you consider that most parents have encouraged their children to continue their educations through college in order to have greater opportunities and get better jobs. Many college students have been led to feel that the world is waiting for them, and when this expectation is not immediately realized, an understandable dejection sets in.

Let your son know that you understand his feelings and sympathize with him in his present situation. Try to impress upon him that while he may not be able to put to direct and immediate use the knowledge he acquired at college, it is nevertheless of great potential value to him. But even though there is a discouraging discrepancy between the job he expected and the reality of the job market today, this does not mean that he and his friends can't create jobs for themselves. The independence they can acquire by forming their *own* organization, rather than working for someone else, may compensate for the disappointment and discouragement they have encountered. I know of some young people in precisely the same situation as your son who literally have become movers; they handle small local jobs, moving furniture, office equipment, and so forth. Other young people I know have learned skills such as furniture refinishing, floor refinishing, and other household repair work.

33

This has provided them not only with a substantial income but also with a sense of fulfillment and an opportunity for expanding their services to include many other people and areas. While your son may seem unmotivated at the present time, perhaps encouragement along these lines will help open new horizons for him.

❦

Working High School Graduate Living with Parents

Our daughter graduated from high school last year and now works as a secretary at a company near our home. Because she is still living with us (she pays a token amount of rent), we feel she should continue to observe our rules about what time she comes in at night. On several occasions recently, she's stayed out with girl friends or dates until the early hours of the morning — and this bothers my husband and me very much. Don't you agree that as long as she lives under our roof, she should observe some sort of curfew?

It's extremely difficult, if not impossible, to enforce rules for someone your daughter's age without damaging communication between you. Theoretically, she is living in *your* house and should abide by *your* rules; at the same time, you must remember that she is growing up, has finished school, and is essentially supporting herself. If, without any discussion, you demand absolute compliance with your regulations, you run the risk of alienating your daughter, who may feel she's being treated like a child. It's far better for you to speak openly with her and let her know how you feel about her late hours — that you are as concerned about her safety as about her activities.

Make it clear that while you don't want to police her life, you do want her to try to be home by midnight (of course recognizing this won't always be possible). Impress upon her that she should respect your parental concern as you respect her maturity and privacy.

If you take the position that she must abide by the house rules or move out, you must be prepared for the possibility that she will do just that. You and your husband might find this a more comfortable solution and might have no hesitation about issuing such an ultimatum. But make sure, before you do, that you're prepared to calmly accept her decision to leave, rather than to respond by acting hurt or angry. Ideally, if maturing young people can maintain open communication with their parents — whether living together or apart — there is a greater chance for developing mutual respect, deeper love, and the marvelous understanding that parents are there when needed as a child attempts to make his or her way in the world.

❦

Adjusting to College

Our seventeen-year-old daughter is a freshman at a college that's a two-hour drive from our home. When she first went away, she was terribly homesick and wanted to come home every weekend. We made arrangements for her to do so, but we thought that as time went by, she'd adjust to her new situation. It has been months now, and she's still "miserable" at school; she comes home every weekend and resists returning to school on Sunday night. What can we do to help? If we forbid her to come home so often, will she think we don't love her?

Many young people have initial difficulties adjusting to college, but they're usually able to adapt to the new environment within a few months. Your daughter is taking longer to adjust, probably because she hasn't had much prior experience being away from home, and also because she may be having some trouble establishing friendships with peers. This can be very difficult. There's tremendous pressure at some colleges, both socially and academically, and she has had to start all over to establish a framework of satisfaction and trust in which she is comfortable — without the support of her family and old friends. Fearing rejection, your daughter may be hesitant about approaching classmates to establish friendships, or she may be uneasy that she will be unable to maintain her grades.

I suggest that you encourage her to go to the student health service at her college and seek out a guidance counselor who works with young students who are having some difficulty adjusting to their new life. Your daughter should have the counsel of someone who is familiar with her new social environment and the pressures it causes. While encouraging her to get this kind of help, assure her that your concern is for her feelings of misery and in no way does this mean she's not welcome in her home whenever she wants to return.

Problems like this should not be taken lightly. Adjusting to college is not an easy task and represents a major transition in the life of young people. Your daughter will have enough pressures at the academic level — some of which can mount up tragically to overwhelm some college students — and she doesn't need more problems on top of it. If she can find satisfaction in her new life, she will be far more comfortable with herself and be freer to explore all the possibilities for her personal growth.

❦

Dreams of Glory and the Drifting High School Graduate

My eighteen-year-old son's been out of high school for about nine months now. He's living at home with us and hasn't taken any steps toward exploring a real career or profession; all he does is talk vaguely about being a "rock star." Are we wrong to let him drift along while he entertains his fantasies that "things will work out" without any effort on his part?

Yes, you are wrong to let him coast along like this. It's important that you let him know that life is not built around "things working out" but that it takes concerted effort on his part to define his goals — even if they are only short-term ones that help him explore possibilities for his future — and make a plan of action for achieving these goals.

I assume that you are supporting your son during this time. This can only encourage him to sit back and fantasize about his successes rather than face the realities required to accomplish them. I don't think you should make skeptical remarks about his being a rock star — that understandably will make him upset and angry. However, you should encourage him to take an active role in his journey to stardom. Urge him to get a job so that he can pay for his lessons, equipment, and everyday expenses, and can even make contributions for his room and board.

Even if he is not working toward a specific goal at this time, he can still work in some capacity to earn sufficient money to assume responsibility for his own care. During that time, he can explore or think through more specific goals for the job or profession he will ultimately want.

Work is a humbling experience that helps people come to terms with the problems of independence and responsibility. If your son doesn't like the work he does but recognizes the fact that he *must* work in order to support himself, he will ultimately become more motivated to work toward something that provides him with greater fulfillment and satisfaction in his everyday activities. But as long as his fantasies are being economically supported by his family, and he is being treated as if he is still dependent, he will not feel the pressures necessary to embark on a course of action. And he will be kept from growing, not only vocationally, but emotionally as well.

❦

Teenage Auto Accident – Paying for the Damage

My sixteen-year-old was in an accident with our car, and the bill for repairs is going to be close to $600. My husband says our son must work to pay for this amount on his own. But I know how sorry our son is, and that he's a good and careful driver — and I know how long this bill will take for him to work off. We could afford to cover the damage on this one — wouldn't it be all right for us to pay the amount this time?

Since your son is remorseful for the accident and is basically a good and careful driver, you should give him some help in restituting the losses caused by his accident. At the same time, it's important for him to recognize and share somewhat in the financial burden for the repairs, but it sounds to me as if he recognizes the gravity of what occurred and is likely to be more careful in the future. In fact, it's possible for your entire family to gain from his unfortunate experience by exercising compassion and understanding in helping him deal with this situation. Instead of your paying the whole amount this time (and we hope the last time), have your son assume responsibility for some part of the $600. If you establish a regular weekly amount that he can pay without extreme sacrifices, he will be able to handle this burden without resentment and at the same time feel that his parents are willing to help him in his difficulties.

If you find in a few months from now that he has been diligent in making these payments and that he continues to drive carefully, you might find it appropriate to waive his remaining financial contributions. This would not undermine his sense of responsibility but would teach him that such problems can be handled with compromise and compassion.

❦

Boys Who Play with Dolls

We have three daughters (ages five, seven, and nine) and a two-year-old son. Our son loves his sisters and spends most of his time with them playing dolls, "house," and so forth. My husband and I wonder if he'll develop any problems because of this.

There is no reason whatsoever to be worried. The important thing is that your son have a good, solid, meaningful relationship based on *his* individuality. As long as his own particular interests and needs are nurtured by the adults around him, his identity as a person, as well as his identity as a male, will emerge spontaneously.

Right now, the pleasure the child gains from playing with his sisters may lead him to engage in their "feminine" play. However, the interests of most children fluctuate, and sooner or later, he — and the girls — may be absorbed instead in baseball or ship models. Boys' playing with dolls should cause no more alarm than girls' playing with toy cars. In fact, the more children's play departs from sex-role stereotypes, the easier they will find it to share the roles and activities they will engage in as grownups and parents later on.

❦

Male – Female Differences

I'm certain that my two-year-old daughter acts more feminine and flirtatious than my rough-and-tumble four-year-old son ever did. Isn't it true that boys and girls behave in certain masculine and feminine ways right from birth?

I would say that, in general, boys and girls do behave differently as a result of their gender, and in some cases these differences are evident at birth. Hormones play an important part in the way emotions are expressed. However, cultural conditioning also plays a very important role in the determination of what is "masculine" and what is "feminine." Certain patterns of behavior are supported or reinforced by our society, while others elicit a negative reaction that serves to suppress them. To complicate things further, genetic factors also play a role in emotions and temperament; people often inherit certain emotional tendencies from their parents and other ancestors.

Some feminists have argued that all emotional differences are culturally determined. While I consider myself a feminist, I cannot deny the dramatic changes in behaviors I've seen in patients who for various reasons have been given male or female hormones as part of their treatment. In particular, when masculine hormones are used to treat patients with certain blood diseases, there is an obvious increase in aggressive behavior. Other differences have emerged in studies done to determine the reactions of male and female children to frustrating situations in the first two years of their lives. The findings of one such study show that male toddlers, when placed in an enclosed area and enticed by an object outside that area, persisted for a substantially longer period of time in trying to reach the desired object. Female toddlers tried for a shorter period of time and then cried out to get help. While some cultural factors may have entered into this behavior, it's unlikely that they could have accounted for all the differences, some of which were clearly along sexual lines.

❦

Teenage Girl Not Interested in Boys

My teenage daughter plays on many school teams, and because of her absorption in these activities, she has little time to pay attention to her appearance or the romantic attention of boys. This distresses both my mother and mother-in-law very much; they are always after me to influence my daughter to be more "feminine." Are they right? Is my daughter's life unbalanced?

You should try to help your daughter achieve her own personal fulfillment and happiness and develop her own unique interests to her fullest potential. At the same time, I see nothing wrong with helping her to appreciate the grooming habits and social graces that will aid her in the years ahead. It's not your job, however, to push her into developing seductive techniques for attracting boys. In time, her interest in those matters will grow, but at the present time she seems to be more fulfilled by her activities than by her contact with the opposite sex. If your daughter is happy, doing well in school, capable of enjoying friendships, and responsive to the emotional demands placed on her, I would say her life seems balanced.

It's difficult for parents who are pressured by "old-fashioned" relatives and friends. When this happens, avoid arguing the pros and cons of any issue, but make it clear to others that ideas about "how boys and girls behave" are changing, and the expectations and interests of your children are changing, too. Thank your relatives for their concern and assure them that you will take their ideas into consideration, and perhaps they'll become more willing to understand your point of view.

❦

Tenderness, Tears, and Masculinity

I've always told my eight-year-old son that it's all right to cry and show his emotions. Yet when I see that the other little boys in the neighborhood are much more "macho," I worry that I'm wrong to encourage my son to behave in a way that might cause him to feel out of place and even be ridiculed.

It's not only correct for parents to encourage children to be sensitive and responsive to other people, it's also important to help children learn to cope with their feelings. No one learns to handle his feelings by repressing them or denying their existence. In my years of practice as a psychologist, I've had to help innumerable people face their deepest feelings and then learn to express them in socially acceptable ways. Tears of sadness or happiness in no way reflect emotional weakness or indicate an inability to compete in the "real world." Emotional sensitivity and the capacity to withstand stress are characteristics that can easily go hand in hand.

Let your child know that some people avoid expressing their feelings because they are afraid of them, and as a cover-up they act "macho" or "cool" or "tough." They think that it seems weak to show their emotions when, in fact, the opposite is often the case. Tell him, however, that other boys might tease him if they see him cry or express his feelings. You might suggest that he hold some of his feelings back temporarily if he's in the company of children who might ridicule him, and wait until he's among friends or family, who are not so threatened by the expression of his emotions. In this way, you will be helping him express his feelings while minimizing the possibility of his being teased or rejected by his peers. It's important to get across the message that it's all right to have feelings, but that you sometimes have to be selective in how and where you express them.

❦

Boys and Baby Care

I asked my five-year-old son if he wanted to help diaper the new baby, and he replied that "Only Mommies take care of babies." Should I encourage him to help?

I feel very strongly that young males, from an early age onward, should be encouraged to participate in all the responsibilities of parenthood. I believe that mothers and fathers should share equally in the responsibilities of raising children — and thereby share in the joys and satisfactions as well.

When your son makes the statement that "Mommies take care of babies," you should tell him that "Daddies should do the same" and then show him ways in which he might help. It will reinforce your position if your husband is willing to help, too. If, at an early age, all children see both mothers and fathers actively involved in feeding, bathing, and changing the baby's diaper, they themselves will be much more inclined to take on that role later in life.

❦

The Restless Sleeper

My energetic eight-year-old is a restless sleeper. He tosses and turns and talks in his sleep, and sometimes he even sits up. Could this active sleep behavior reflect tension or anxiety, or is it merely a normal aspect of his lively nature?

The sleeping habits of children are almost as varied as children themselves. Some are such sound sleepers that they are not even awakened by a full bladder, and wet the bed. Other children are such light sleepers that whispers from a nearby room are enough to awaken them.

Real disturbances in sleep, however, are frequently an indication of underlying emotional problems or environmental tensions. We all know that when the pressures mount and worries increase, sleeplessness prevails, or other disruptions in one's rest may occur. Instead of refreshing sleep, a person's mind may be filled with thoughts of the day's unfinished business or uneasiness about anticipated events.

Sleep has been the subject of a great deal of research and investigation. Some theorists have concluded that dreaming is our means of trying to resolve some of the day's actual unfinished problems, as well as problems persisting from the past in the unconscious mind. Another recent theory is that dream activity is in some way a process of "dumping" unnecessary mental information that frees the mind to take on other challenges.

In this particular case, if your child's active sleep behavior is indeed due to tension or anxiety, his emotional state would reflect itself in other ways as well. During his daytime activities, you would notice other signs of tension and unhappiness. If, however, he is a happy child who gets along with other children, does well in school, and appears well rested even after what appears to be restless sleep, in all likelihood his sleep patterns are simply a normal extension of his active daytime personality.

❦

Helping an Infant in Pain

My ten-month-old son has had recurrent ear infections since he was three months of age. We are coping with the situation medically, and our son receives proper medication and regular check-ups, so my concern is for his emotional health. He is in a good deal of pain when he gets the infection, and although I do everything possible to comfort him, many times I am unsuccessful. I am afraid that his situation may harm him psychologically and lead to his mistrust of me in the future. He seems to look at me as though he thinks I should be taking away his pain, and I am not. Could our relationship be harmed by this?

While persistent, intense pain is indeed unpleasant for any child, your son need not develop emotional problems because of it. Most children can *feel* the sincere compassion of the parents who are trying to comfort them. Even though it may not be possible for you to take away the hurt, your child knows that you are trying. As hard as it may be for you to see him so upset, hold him, cuddle him, and try to be with him during his episodes of pain.

Some doctors recommend that you should leave a child alone at such times; they feel that there is nothing you can do about it anyway and that the child will associate the pain with the person present during it and will therefore develop resentment toward the parent on hand. I disagree with that notion wholeheartedly. In my years of work with hospitalized and ill children, I have had a great deal of experience with these situations, and I find that in such circumstances the relationships may even become stronger and better ones. If a child who has been through substantial pain or illness has also had a parent there to consistently offer comfort and support, the child will become even more convinced of that parent's love and compassion. In fact, the feeling of trust grows rather than diminishes.

❧

Physical Complaints — Real or Psychological

My ten-year-old often wakes up in the morning and says she doesn't feel well — her "head hurts" or her "tummy aches." But unless children obviously have a fever, how can a parent tell whether they are faking or not? And if she is faking, why might my daughter be doing this? Is there a psychological explanation? I hate to insist she go to school if she's really ill, yet she seems to conveniently feel "sick" whenever something comes up that she doesn't feel like doing.

When you look for "psychological explanations," in all likelihood you can find them. Many people psychologize about everything in life and sometimes fail to see some of the more direct, logical, and uncomplicated reasons for why something is happening. All "normal" people face daily pressures, encounter losses, endure anxieties, and suffer traumas; the person who overpsychologizes is apt to seize on these normal problems as the "cause" for everything, including physical complaints. You can be sure that I am *not* trying to demean the importance of emotional factors in everyday life, but I am simply cautioning you against jumping to psychological conclusions and ignoring other possible explanations for an event.

If your child has frequent complaints of physical discomfort, even if they seem to be precipitated by major or minor stresses, it's essential that you have her checked out medically by a physician. In my professional experience I have encountered many children with real physical problems that had been incorrectly diagnosed as psychosomatic or psychogenic. You owe it to your child to explore fully any physical basis for her aches and pains.

Concurrently, I think it is important for you to find out what is happening in her life that might be causing her to develop symptoms and complaints like these. Frequently a child who is bullied by another child, intimidated by a teacher, or rejected by her peer group might find things sufficiently unpleasant to develop anxiety or depression, both of which have physical counterparts and come out in physical symptoms. If she is intensely anxious, this can create a *real* headache and a *real* stomachache. In fact, some children become nauseated and even vomit in response to being forced into an unpleasant situation.

If you find no possible explanation for her symptoms after a medical examination and an evaluation of her environment, you then have to deal with the problem by making it clear to her that life consists of many demands, commitments, and responsibilities that are not always easy or pleasant. Point out to her that she is simply going to have to pull herself together and get on with her routine. Don't be harsh or punitive — be firm

47

and matter-of-fact in your attitude — and let her know that you are standing by to help her cope in any way you can. One of life's most important lessons is learning how to take in stride all the dull, uninteresting, and sometimes unpleasant elements that are part of one's life. Now is an important time for you to help your daughter work out a positive approach toward dealing with these situations.

❦

Sickness as an Excuse

My eight-year-old often says he "doesn't feel well" or "has a stomachache" just before he has to leave for school or do an errand for me. I think he's just trying to get out of doing things that are unpleasant, so I usually play down his "sickness" and send him on his way, even though he goes off saying how "mean" I am. Sometimes I worry, though, that I'm doing the wrong thing. Should I react in a different way to his complaints?

It's not unusual for anyone, children included, to "feel bad" when faced with a stressful situation. Stomachaches are often very real pains that develop when a person is faced not only with unpleasantness but with frustrating situations that are an inescapable part of life. We live in a culture that offers little acceptable opportunity for avoiding upsetting experiences other than through illness. For this reason, people may actually become ill as a way of avoiding unpleasant events.

Parents who are very protective of their children sometimes overreact to a child's physical complaints. This overreaction can lead to a greater tendency for a child to feign illness in order to gain attention or avoid unpleasantness and challenging situations. I believe it's best for parents to take a somewhat matter-of-fact attitude when the initial complaints are voiced and not to react in an extreme fashion one way or another as they try to evaluate a child's symptoms. Ideally, it's best to have a doctor check your son at the time he complains of illness, but this is not always possible or practical. As a general rule, I suggest that you take your child's temperature. If your son doesn't have a fever, acknowledge that you know he feels uncomfortable, but since he doesn't have a fever, he'll just have to go to school. While it is a calculated risk to send a child with physical complaints off to school, you have to weigh this against the effects that such a pattern of behavior may have on the child in the long run.

In my experience, I have found that when children are under stress in school because of heavy work loads or upcoming examinations for which the child is unprepared or an overbearing teacher, reports of illness often occur. If your child complains frequently about aches and pains, you should unquestionably see a physician and have the doctor perform whatever tests are medically advisable. You should also investigate the reasons that may underlie a child's stress and anxiety.

I don't believe in being "mean" to children under any circumstances, nor do I suggest that you ignore their complaints. If they are indeed ill on school days, I think you should see to their needs and make them as comfortable as possible — but avoid at all costs making this an enjoyable and special event. I advise against letting children watch television during the hours they would otherwise be in school, and feel that it's best for them to rest and sleep instead. If they seem capable of engaging in an activity, have them do schoolwork. Contact the school and find out what your son's assignments are and what work is being done during the time he misses school. If he feels sufficiently well to want to do something, have him read or do schoolwork. In this way, you're holding your child responsible for his regular tasks and at the same time showing concern for his feelings and needs. The main thing is that you not reward illness in a way that encourages your child to use it as an excuse for getting out of situations he'd rather avoid.

❦

Adolescent Preoccupation with Sickness and Death

Lately my sixteen-year-old daughter has become fearful of contracting some serious illness. She's perfectly healthy, and athletic too, but she worries about dying from cancer or a sudden stroke or even a heart attack! Is this a common worry for a healthy teenager? Why is she worrying about such things? How can I reassure her?

While teenagers do tend to be a bit more preoccupied with their bodies during their transition from childhood to adulthood, your daughter's worries seem to be somewhat more extreme. When a healthy and athletic young person has such fears of death or serious illness, it generally reflects some underlying conflict. Sometimes guilt about certain thoughts or impulses leads a person to develop excessive fears. These fears, in a sense, represent "forbidden" ideas or impulses that have been repressed. The feelings then are displaced externally into fear of cancer, stroke, heart attack, or death. Although it's not totally unrealistic to be fearful of these, her fears do seem out of proportion to reality. It's precisely their extreme nature that suggests something is going on beneath the surface that she is unable to express.

You should certainly offer her as much reassurance as you can that she is young and healthy and unlikely to be stricken by these afflictions — but generally in such a situation, this doesn't help much. Suggest to her that perhaps there are thoughts on her mind that make her uncomfortable and cause her to be particularly anxious and sensitive about everything. Give her the opportunity of speaking with you about these thoughts and feelings, but don't pressure her. Let her know that if she's unable to discuss with you what's bothering her, you will help her find a doctor who is trained to help people with their fears. She may deny that she has any problems and reject any offerings of help. If so, tell her that you know it must be hard to live with fears and anxieties such as hers and that it's terrible for a young and healthy person to be so uncomfortable. Stress that it *is* possible for her to overcome and learn to deal with such fears.

❦

Physical Reactions to Stress

It seems that before tests or trips or the first day of school, or any other challenging experiences, my eleven-year-old will announce she "feels sort of weird" and mope around as though she's sick. There are never any other physical signs — the doctor says she's fine — so I'm not always sympathetic and send her off to whatever it is she says she feels "too funny" to do. What should my tactics be in handling this? What do you think she's up to? Is she pretending, or does she really indeed feel the way she says she does?

I see no reason whatsoever for you to doubt that she "really feels the way she says she does." The episodes that seem to cause her to have these "weird feelings" are situations of uncertainty. They are understandably stressful experiences, and stress causes various physical changes such as an increased heartbeat, sweaty palms, dryness of the mouth, and sometimes even a feeling of weakness and strange sensations in the stomach. While she may mope around as though she's sick, she is having a physical and mental reaction to stress. I think you are doing the right thing when you send her off to do whatever she says makes her feel "funny." However, offer her support and encouragement as well. Let her know you understand why she feels the way she does, and at the same time let her know she'll get through it all right and feel better as soon as she gets into the experience. Your support can go a long way toward helping her master these disquieting feelings and can lead to the development of greater emotional strength, which she can call forth the next time that feeling of "weirdness" overtakes her. As a general rule, these feelings diminish over time, particularly with parental support. Even if she doesn't overcome this discomfort completely when faced with challenging experiences, you needn't fear as long as she is not so immobilized or frightened that she can't cope effectively with the challenges she faces.

❦

Fear or Phobia

My twenty-eight-year-old sister gets terribly claustrophobic in elevators, even to the point that it's impossible for her to ride in them. I have phobias about spiders and let out a shriek if I even sight one. What causes such phobias to develop and hang on like this? What do they represent? How should I explain phobias to my children, who see that their aunt and mother are in terror about these things? And how do you keep your children from picking up such fears themselves?

A phobia is basically a severe anxiety reaction set off by certain objects or situations that realistically cause little or no actual danger — yet a person's response can be irrational, overwhelming, and can cause intense and crippling anxiety. It is true that some fears are somewhat appropriate and not without a certain basis in fact. After all, on occasion people do get stuck in elevators, and sometimes spiders do bite and that bite can be poisonous. However, these fears can grow out of all proportion, and a real problem sets in when anxiety over these things becomes incapacitating. If your sister was not able to move freely in circumstances where elevator travel was essential, or if you became fearful of working about your house or going outdoors because you might encounter a spider, the problems would be severely crippling.

Occasionally phobias develop following a real-life experience, such as falling from a horse or being in an automobile accident. Usually they are not set off by a literal experience, but have a rather deep psychological significance. Phobias result because a person at some time or other had a very strong impulse to express a feeling or do something that was highly unacceptable to his or her conscience. In an attempt to place distance between oneself and that "forbidden" impulse, the human mind reacts with a series of emotional mechanisms. The mind represses the impulse altogether and does its best to deny that it even happened, or blames it on someone or something else (It wasn't me, it was that "bad monster under my bed") or takes the person toward whom that unacceptable impulse was meant and displaces those feelings onto something else. ("It's not my mother who creates this terrifying feeling in me, it's an animal or an insect or being enclosed in small spaces.") The phobia is to some extent the end product of all the intricate psychological mechanisms that people use to protect themselves from expressing an unacceptable impulse toward someone they love or depend on. In general, once established, phobias persist and sometimes get worse as those repressed impulses continue to build up. If this happens, professional psychological help is essential. Some people are successful in facing their phobias squarely and mobilizing their resources to overcome their fears. Others develop what we call counterphobias and go to the opposite extreme to engage in the very activities that cause their anxiety. People with a fear of high places may become mountain climbers, others may force themselves into contact with creatures that terrify them. In this way, a person gains active mastery over something that formerly had caused a great deal of panic and discomfort.

In explaining your fears to your children, tell them that everyone at some time or another is frightened of various things or situations. Point out that frequently these fears are irrational but that it's hard to stop them simply by talking yourself out of it. For the most part, such fears are not "contagious." Children will not pick up a specific phobia from parents or relatives unless the children have certain underlying emotional weaknesses themselves. On the other hand, they can develop some anxiety when they see a parent panic, since children need to feel that their parents have sufficient stability and control to help *them* with their fears and problems.

❦

Inconsistent Discipline

My husband sets up rules that our children are supposed to follow, then he turns around and allows them to break the rules "just this once." For instance, he told the older kids they have a curfew, but one night when they were late, he laughed and acted as if it didn't matter, only to get very angry the next night when they did the very same thing. Isn't it harmful to the children when rules are enforced on some days and ignored on others?

It certainly is — in fact, it makes things difficult for everyone in the family. In a situation like this, most children become increasingly anxious because they never know what to expect. Moreover, it causes them to break rules frequently in an attempt to find out what the rules and regulations actually are. Believe it or not, children *want* rules, provided they are allowed some range of freedom. Children usually feel more protected when their parents are consistent and reasonable in setting up and maintaining appropriate rules.

In all likelihood, your children have some inner doubts about their trust in your husband. His inconsistency causes these doubts, and perhaps even some resentment. Children have often told me, "I wish my parents would stick to what they say; I never know whether to believe them or not." Parents sometimes think that if they are flexible — as your husband probably thinks he is being — their children will think they are democratic and generous. The opposite is true.

While compromise and understanding are necessary in the enforcement of rules, meaningless inconsistency is not. If rules are changed for children because of special circumstances, reasons should be given and discussed in advance, if possible. But if there are no guidelines whatsoever to explain a parent's unpredictable pronouncements, only confusion and resentment can result.

❦

Fixed Bedtime

Is it necessary that every young child have a fixed bedtime hour? My two-year-old daughter has never seemed to need as much sleep as other children; she gave up taking an afternoon nap months ago, and lately has even rebelled at going to bed at

8:00 P.M. I do not wish to be a rigid parent; on the other hand, I feel some rules are necessary; a child "needs" a certain amount of sleep a night, doesn't she?

Children's needs can vary greatly. Research has shown that some children literally require a great deal of sleep, while others seem to need very little in order to function adequately. Moreover, observations show that children with this lesser sleep need develop just as well as, and in many cases faster than, children who have a greater need for sleep.

It is hard to force children to go to sleep when they are not tired. In fact, such haggling makes bedtime an unpleasant event. I suggest you be as flexible as possible and adapt your daughter's schedule to better fit her needs. If she does not tend to become sleepy until nine o'clock, your insistence that she go before that time can only serve to frustrate her unnecessarily. If she feels the need to have a light on and play with her toys for a while to help her relax, don't hesitate to let her do this. (Most two-year-olds like to have a parent read to them until they drift off to sleep naturally and comfortably.)

I agree that rules are necessary in raising children, but sometimes a rigid bedtime can make sleep a time of conflict rather than a time of comfort. My experience has indicated that parents who insist on an early, unchanging bedtime for children do so for their own convenience, in order to get the children out of the way. I am sympathetic toward parents, who do indeed need to have time for themselves, but putting children to bed before they are ready can cause more problems than it will solve.

❧

Responsibility for Care of Pets

*Our boys, six and eight, begged for a puppy, and my husband
and I finally agreed. But we made the boys promise they would
be the ones to take care of a pet, and if they didn't, the dog
would have to go. Well, six months have passed, and although
the boys love the dog, I'm the one who ends up feeding and
disciplining it. I now feel that we should follow through on our
original threat and give the dog away. Do you agree? Or did we
handle this in the wrong way from the very start?*

Frankly speaking, you should not have allowed the situation
to deteriorate over so long a period. You should have monitored
their promise on a daily basis and consistently enforced the
rules you originally set up. Allowing yourself to be drawn into
assuming the responsibility of caring for the dog played a very
important part in creating the problem you are faced with
now.

What you and your husband must do is to sit down quietly
with your children in a setting where there are no distractions.
Let the boys know you have a very serious matter to deal with
and that a very important decision has to be made. Speak
calmly and firmly, and if the boys seem shocked or stunned at
the businesslike atmosphere, you'll know you are on the right
track. Make it clear that their pet is about to be given up for
adoption. Explain that you have reached this decision after
careful evaluation of the situation and want to place the matter
before them to see if they have any other suggestions that will
be acceptable to you. Have ready in the back of your mind a
suggestion that *is* acceptable — one that gives back to the boys
the primary responsibility for caring for their pet — and be
absolutely prepared to play your part in firmly enforcing this
policy. This meeting should not be allowed to disintegrate into
an argument or digress into other matters that detract from
your main point. It's precisely a businesslike kind of atmos-

phere that will convey the seriousness of the issue and, hopefully, will lead to a plan that preserves the integrity of your household and all the family members, including the puppy.

❦

Defiance in Children

I tell my child to straighten up his room, he races out to play; I ask him to be nice to his little sister, he deliberately takes a swing at her. What does it mean when a child seems to always do the opposite of what you ask? We've tried berating him and punishing him to no avail.

Most normal children defy parental wishes from time to time; it's an expression of their individuality and quest for independence. In addition, there are certain ages at which children are particularly defiant. Two-year-olds and adolescents head this list, with four-year-olds following closely behind.

I suspect that a child who totally complies with all parental wishes on all occasions has certain emotional problems. However, when a child *always* does the opposite of what you ask, this too seems to reflect a disturbance in the parent-child relationship. Children who totally defy your every wish are telling you how angry they are, how resentful of your authority. For the most part, they think you have ignored their feelings or have misused your power in your relationship with them. Unfortunately, some parents either ignore their children or hound them with criticism. They evidence little or no interest in a child's accomplishments or pleasures. They are sometimes overly punitive and often inconsistent with their rules and regulations. If interaction with children consists of such factors, almost any comment, request, or wish expressed by parents will elicit a resentful, critical, and negativistic response.

If you are caught up in a situation like this, you have to make a careful reassessment of your relationship with your child. This can best be done with professional help. It's not an easy task to undertake, and you cannot expect positive results overnight. Nevertheless, it is the best approach and one that will ultimately lead you closer to the kind of relationship you always wished you could have with your son.

❧

Spanking and Physical Punishment

I've read about the law in Sweden that forbids parents from striking their children or treating them in "humiliating ways." What sort of effect will this have on children who are never spanked or given a slap for misbehavior? Can you shed any light on the motivations of these legislators? Do you understand or agree with the ideas behind what they're doing?

Anyone knowledgeable in the field of child psychology knows that spanking or physical punishment not only has no beneficial effects for a child but can be psychologically harmful. Swedish legislators, who have been made aware of this information by child-development experts, have been appropriately responsive. They have outlawed spanking and other humiliating ways of punishing children, including the withholding of meals as a punishment.

Basically, the Swedish law represents a statement by that country of its attitudes toward children. I'm sure there is no intent to put a parent in jail for spanking a child — in fact, no penalties have been set by the legislators for violating this law. And a Swedish child would hardly be likely to actually prosecute a parent. Nevertheless, it speaks well for the humane instincts of the Swedish people, who have sufficiently strong feelings about the integrity of their children to pass a law protecting their self-esteem and dignity.

Few of us, if any, can look back upon being spanked or slapped without remembering a feeling of resentment and a desire to retaliate. Spanking establishes a pattern in which physical violence, as slight as it may be, is considered an acceptable means of controlling the behavior of others. To me this is amoral and sets the stage for more violent activity later on.

Proponents of spanking claim that it "straightens children out" and "gets them to do what you want." While it indeed may get children to "behave" or "perform" at that particular moment, in the long run it can have no positive effects. I'm convinced that every child or young person who becomes destructive and hostile toward figures or institutions of authority is retaliating in some way against a parent or parent surrogate who brutalized the child in some physical way in the past.

❦

Discipline and Punishment of Teenagers

My husband tries to rigidly enforce the rule that our fifteen-year-old son be home by midnight on weekends. Again and again our son comes in later than that, and again and again there are terrible fights. How do we resolve this?

If you clamp down on teenagers and try to make them stick to strict rules, as your husband does, you're bound to create resentment and perhaps outright defiance. Besides that, it's impossible to police your son twenty-four hours a day, and there's virtually no punishment you can enforce that would do more than intensify the anger between your son and your husband.

Situations like this require open communication and mutual understanding. I encourage parents to let their teenagers know that they *are* aware of their children's increased need to do things on their own. But stress that it's not easy for parents to simply let children go off on their own without any rules or guidelines. Emphasize that it's not their irresponsibility that upsets or worries you, but in certain situations you are concerned about the possible dangers that could come up. Let them know you are *not* trying to restrict or control them, but simply want some peace of mind about their whereabouts and activities. Explain to your son that if he's not home by midnight, or by whatever hour you mutually agree on, you begin to worry. Urge him to try to make the deadline you all agree upon. Let him know that you can understand that there are times when it might not be possible for him to be home precisely on time, but that you'd like him to call and let you know something has come up. With compromise and understanding on your part, you can at least be in communication rather than at war with your teenager.

If your son continues to violate or take advantage of agreements you make on matters such as this, let him know that it disappoints you and makes it more difficult for you to allow the freedom you want to give him. Even then, don't take a harsh or punitive position as this simply will cause him to "dig in" even more firmly on his side. The greater the understanding and acceptance on your part, the easier it will be for him to "give in" and respect your feelings and wishes.

I know that many parents might disagree with me, feeling that unless you severely punish teenagers for their violations, you are condoning unacceptable behavior. But my experience tells me that severe punishments or rigid rules not only provoke more rebelliousness but that young people frequently retaliate by developing a negative and self-defeating attitude toward *all* rules and regulations that come up later in their lives.

❦

Children's "Greediness" at Christmas

Every year, my children (ages seven, ten, and thirteen) make up a Christmas list that would boggle the budget of a Rockefeller. They list endless toys that they've seen and want, and act disappointed if they don't get them all. I feel upset about this — we have nice kids whose desire for "more more more" seems to be out of character. Is it right for them to want so many things? Is there reason for me to be alarmed about what seems to be their excessive greediness?

To me, this does not represent "greediness" but is a reaction to the excitement, the indulgence, and the departure from the constraints that adults attempt to exercise throughout the rest of the year. Festive foods and beverages are consumed in more than normal quantities, sometimes parties are held, friends visit — and the scope of our wishes and desires is also extended.

And since Christmas is so focused on children, they are even more intensely stimulated along these lines. Toys and gifts for children are widely advertised, and in a very tantalizing way. Their temptations are increased as everyone asks them, "What do you want for Christmas?" For a child this is mind-boggling — and would also be budget-boggling if parents were to fulfill all their wishes. The disappointment they feel after their presents have been opened is more because the gift giving has come to an end than because they did not get all they wanted. I don't think you have to be defensive or make moralistic judgments when you see this disappointment, or what appears to be their greed. The disappointment is simply due to reentry into the "normal world" of all the un-Christmasy days ahead.

Let your children know that you understand that "it would be great if this could continue all year — but it can't, and that's simply the way it is." Give them a smile of encouragement to carry them through their letdown and set a note of optimism for the year to come.

❦

The Truth About Santa Claus

Once before you talked about Santa Claus. You said it was harmful for adults to perpetuate his myth to their children. I can't believe you haven't gotten some adverse reaction about your stand. Do you still feel so strongly about Santa?

I have caused some commotion by airing my views on Santa Claus, but most of it has resulted from a misunderstanding about what I was saying. I'm not at all against perpetuating the *myth* of Santa. In fact, that's precisely what I favor. A *myth* is a story passed down from generation to generation, or as Webster's dictionary puts it, "a person or thing existing only in imagination." I'm not opposed to the myth; I'm opposed to telling children that Santa Claus is real. And then, building on this basic untruth, most parents compound the problem even further by continuing to lie about how Santa can get around to so many places in such a short time or what happens if a house has no chimney. Ultimately, when a child learns the truth, trust in his or her parents can be seriously undermined.

While I don't recommend stopping youngsters as they walk down the street and telling them that "Santa Claus is a fake," I do reaffirm my position that children should be told the truth about Santa Claus when they ask if he is real. Tell a child that Santa is a make-believe character, but that even grownups like to pretend he is real during Christmas time. Children are eminently capable of enjoying such fantasies and sometimes find even greater satisfaction in these than in reality.

❧

Christmas and the Disappointed Child

Our daughter desperately wants something for Christmas that we can't afford. Several weeks ago, our eight-year-old saw an elaborate and expensive dollhouse in a store — and from that moment on, she's talked of nothing else but finding that doll-house under the tree on Christmas morning. Her heart's never been so set on anything in her life, but the house is altogether out of the question for us financially. Should we tell her sternly we don't want to hear another word about this, or should we let her go on until Christmas morning and hope she'll be distracted by her other presents? Will a great disappointment like this be harmful to her emotionally?

I certainly don't think you should flatly forbid her to talk about wanting the dollhouse, nor do I think you should simply let her fantasize without a word from you until Christmas morning. By handling the situation in either of these ways, you make your daughter even more vulnerable to disappointment and are sidestepping an opportunity to help her learn to cope with one of the most important realities in life — the fact that we cannot always have what we want no matter how much we want it.

It's essential that you make it clear to your daughter that you understand how strong her feelings are about this dollhouse, but that the cost is much more than you can possibly afford. Suggest alternative presents that are within your means. If her heart is as set on this dollhouse as you say, in all likelihood nothing else will do. Nevertheless, by offering her options, you are showing her that you care about her feelings, are willing to do what you can to give her something she likes, and at the same time are preparing her for the disappointment she will feel when she ultimately realizes the dollhouse will not be hers. While she may continue to insist that the house will indeed appear, on Christmas morning she'll remember that you told the truth. And by telling her the truth, you are in a far better position to help her deal with whatever emotional distress may occur at the time, as well as on other occasions throughout her life.

No, I don't think this "great disappointment" will harm her emotionally. In fact, I believe if she is properly prepared, and made to understand why her wish is not possible, the reality of the situation can help her develop a more realistic and mature outlook on life. As I have said over and over again, you must be honest with your children, prepare them as best you can for what you know will or will not happen, and give them emotional support for dealing with their feelings realistically.

❦

Dealing with Christmas Commercialism

*We grownups are aware of just how much Christmas has
become commercialized, but how do you convey this to your
children? My son and daughter are now five and seven, and I
wonder if they are able to understand the true meaning of the
holidays. How do you explain to children about the real spirit
of the continuity and celebration of the season — whatever your
ethnic or religious commitments/beliefs/background may be? If
things have gotten out of hand, how do you "scale things down"
so there is less mayhem and materialism?*

Unquestionably, everyone must deal with rampant commercialism at Christmas time. Children are especially enticed by
store displays and magazine and television advertising, and by
adults asking them what they want for Christmas. But adults
may become caught up in this as well. Before becoming critical
of your children, it is important to examine your own attitude
and behavior carefully to see if you yourself succumb to the
commercialism of the season. If, for instance, they see you
using the holiday season as a "payoff time" where business
associates or random acquaintances are given gifts reluctantly
or without any thought whatsoever, your children can't help
but view gifts in a materialistic way.

It's extremely difficult for parents to stem the tide of holiday
commercialism, but I believe it can be done by setting an
example for your children and living what you believe. If you
see the holidays as a time for celebrating, sharing, and exchanging tokens of real affection, you can do it in a way that doesn't
require endless sums of money. As your children see you baking
those special cookies that Uncle Fred likes, or planning a gift
subscription to your sister-in-law's favorite magazine, or fram-
ing a school drawing that Grandma admired, they will come to
understand that it's the thoughtfulness behind the gift that will
convey the most meaning to the person receiving it. In this way,

it is possible to let your children know that the size or cost of a gift has no bearing whatsoever on the feelings with which it is given.

As far as tradition is concerned, children love it and sometimes get more caught up in it than adults do. Accounts of the "old days" can have a vivid and intense meaning for children. Reading stories, telling them about your own childhood, and passing on the recollections of your parents and grandparents serve to maintain the continuity of the spirit and meaning of your own background and beliefs. Children of any age can understand this as long as parents themselves *feel* this way and express their feelings with sincerity.

If the holiday season is a meaningful experience for you and your family, if it is one that involves understanding, love, and the expression of thoughtfulness for others, your children will be at least partially "immunized" against commercialism.

❦

Teaching Children to Share at Christmas

Our children's rooms are filled to overflowing with toys, and this year their letters to Santa are more outrageous than ever, filled with endless requests for even more dolls and games and playthings. Last night my husband tossed down one of these letters in despair, poured forth his feelings of cynicism about the whole season, and announced that this year the mounds of presents would be drastically reduced — each child would get one "big" gift and no more. I agree with him that we need to keep things in perspective, but is this the way to do it? Does a great flood of gifts throw children off balance emotionally?

If you and your husband have customarily filled your children's endless requests to Santa Claus, you have created the problem yourself. At this point, it's not fair to abruptly change the situation and in effect punish your children for something that is not their fault. I don't blame them for their endless requests for gifts when they feel they all come from an impersonal figure whose workshop is loaded to the brim. Furthermore, if they believe that Santa "knows if you've been bad or good," the sudden cutoff of presents can be not only a terrible shock but might be seen as an indication of their "badness" as well.

If, however, your children recognize that *real people* are the ones who give the presents, and if you convey to them the real spirit behind sharing and exchanging gifts, you will find it far easier to get things in realistic perspective.

Instead of you and your husband expressing your feelings by curtailing presents so abruptly, apply your feelings in a more positive way. Have your children go through all their playthings and pick out not only those they might have outgrown but perhaps some that they like very much and feel other children might enjoy equally. Suggest that they clean up these toys and give them to some community organization that distributes them to children who are not likely to get gifts otherwise. Don't simply gather the toys yourself, but have your children participate fully in this whole process — and have *them* make the presentation to the charitable organization so they can gain the recognition that generally comes with this kind of sharing and generosity. After all, this might be a good way for your children to learn for themselves who Santa Claus really is. By being little Santas themselves, they should come to understand that *real people* are the ones who give the presents.

❦

Christmas Letdown

Christmas is always a busy, exciting time in our home, but every year I can foresee the letdown that will occur the day after Christmas. (Last year I found my eight-year-old sobbing because "Christmas wasn't there any more," and even my teenagers seem down in the dumps and disgruntled.) Is it natural for my kids to react in such a way? How can you adequately prepare your family for the post-Christmas letdown?

It's absolutely normal for a child — or anyone, for that matter — to feel a letdown following a period of excitement. For some people, the end of the holidays may be a relief — these are people whose holidays may have been lonely or the source of family tension or simply a period of exhaustion in which they attempted to do too much during a short period of time. But for most people, the days before Christmas are a period of happy anticipation. Things build to an exciting pitch, especially for children, and then seem to come to an end very abruptly. Understandably, children are disappointed and might even wish there were "more presents to open" or that "Christmas would be every day of the year." This is not due to greed, it is simply an appropriate reaction to the end of the excitement.

There's no way of preventing or preparing for the disappointment; you've simply got to deal with it when it occurs by offering understanding and emotional support, along with a hug. It's the best way to get back to normal after the holidays.

❦

The Jewish Child and Christmas

We're the only Jewish family in our immediate neighborhood (in which we have many friends), and our children, who are five and eight, can't understand why they, too, can't have a tree and all the toys and trappings that fill the homes of all their playmates at Christmas time. They beg and beg to have a Christmas tree — but when our parents heard we were even considering such a thing, they were so shocked and horrified that we dropped the subject immediately. I love my heritage and want to preserve it, but at the same time I wonder if it's psychologically damaging for our children to feel so "left out" and "different" at this time of the year. How do we explain this to our children? Or should we give in and do what our neighbors do?

There's nothing psychologically damaging about feeling different, but it certainly can hurt to feel left out. Your plight is a very common one for Jewish parents during the Christmas season. Looking at it from a child's viewpoint, beautifully decorated Christmas trees with toys, decorations, sweets, and packages are extremely intriguing, and it is hard to see why other children have the fun of all this when they do not.

While the Christmas tree may symbolize a different religion to you, it doesn't necessarily have any religious significance at all to your children. The wish to have a Christmas tree with piles of toys underneath it is an understandable desire for any child. Many Jewish people feel a Christmas tree represents more the season of the year than a religious belief different from their own, and therefore have no conflict at all about celebrating Hanukkah and having a tree at the same time.

Others, however, think it's hypocritical and feel a strong need to separate themselves from any kind of Christmas symbol. If you feel this way, make your Hanukkah celebration as festive as possible and accompany it with an abundance of foods, gifts, songs, dances, and all else that makes this a meaningful and enjoyable celebration for your children.

Invite your children's friends, as well as your own friends and neighbors who may be Christian, to join in your celebrations. By doing so, you will be sharing with them an experience that goes back many thousands of years. The lives of everyone will be enriched in this way. And on a personal level, your children will be less inclined to feel isolated and more able to be proud that their family is contributing something special to the season.

As friends and families of different faiths interact, they develop a better understanding of how others celebrate their holidays and learn that, despite differences, there is a common spirit that is shared at this time of the year. By marking your celebrations with a sense of pride, you will make the holidays such a positive experience for your children that they will look forward to these events with eager anticipation year after year.

❧

Christmas in the Tropics

Two years ago we moved from the North to a southern state where there's no snow — we have sand and cactus instead. To my surprise, my children and I took this very hard. Now that December is here again, my children are upset because it "isn't like Christmas," and they're very sad and droopy. I share their feelings, too! Is it healthy for us to be longing for the "old" Christmas so that our "new" one is ruined?

There is absolutely nothing wrong with treasuring memories of the past. Our traditions bring us a feeling of pleasure and stability and provide us with something to transmit to our children. At the same time, people may sometimes be so caught up in their old images of how things "used to be" that it is hard for them to accept the possibility of something different but equally rewarding. Different situations can bring different satisfactions — and this applies to "traditional" holidays as well.

Nonetheless, any change from established tradition frequently causes us to feel somewhat jolted. This seems to be what has happened to you and your children. Needless to say, there are many people who live in tropical climates who have become accustomed to Christmas without snow and evergreens. While this is hardly reassuring to you at the moment, you may find that as time goes by, you will adapt to Christmas in your new environment. Encourage your children to look at the fun of finding new ways to celebrate. With your guidance, they can come to look at their new Christmas as an adventure and can concentrate on the excitement of new experiences instead of sadness at the loss of old ones.

If you find after this year that you still can't enjoy the holidays where you are, you might consider planning your next Christmas vacation farther north and in an environment similar to the one you've been used to over the years.

❦

Grown Child Missing the Family Christmas

For years, our whole family has celebrated the holidays together. Now, for the first time, my oldest son, who is twenty and a junior at college, has announced that instead of coming home for the holidays, he's going to go skiing in Colorado with friends. I'm crushed. Is it natural for children all of a sudden to want to be away from their family for the holidays? Does this mean something has been lacking, that Christmas hasn't been as wonderful as I've thought it was? Should I insist that he come home with the rest of us? I really feel wounded and upset about this.

I can understand that you feel distressed about this, since his plans represent a major departure from what you've done over the years as a family. I don't think you should insist that he come home to be with the rest of the family as he's always done, but I think you should let him know that you are upset and that it would have given everyone a feeling of happiness if he could have shared the holidays with them. Urge him to consider a compromise arrangement whereby he spends part of the holiday with you and then joins his friends for the remainder.

However, the fact that he wants to be with his friends does not mean that you are not a closely knit family or that something serious is lacking in his family life. It's simply that many young people, as they get older, spend more and more time with friends during the holidays. Ski resorts are filled with young college people at that time of the year. It's important for you to recognize that your son is becoming independent and that he's moving farther out into the world and gradually creating a life of his own.

I don't think that you should attempt to make him feel intensely guilty about his choice, but I see no harm in letting him know how much you will all miss him. Let him know how joyous it would be for everyone if Christmas could be maintained as the traditional time for the family to be together.

Even if he goes through with his plans, in all likelihood he will have a feeling of nostalgia and may even feel homesick when the holidays arrive. In fact, he will probably miss you as much as you miss him, which may very well lead him to cherish spending Christmas with his family all the more.

❦

ASK DR. SALK

Dreading the Holiday Season

I work so hard to make Christmas a joyous time every year. I do my best to buy gifts that are right for everyone, to decorate, and to prepare big meals. But somehow, no matter how I try to keep my spirits up, I actually dread the holidays. And then I feel guilty that I dread them. What's going on here? Why am I in such a state over a time that should be so wonderful?

The holiday season is a time of intense emotional excitement. Most people anticipate the holidays with great feelings of exhilaration and happiness because it is the time when work schedules are relaxed and people gather together with friends and relatives to eat and drink and celebrate. It seems obvious that you have had the burden of handling the preparations in your family, and, understandably, your anticipation of the holiday season is not pleasant because it means increasing responsibilities. As each year passes, you remember more of the burdens and less of the happiness. This seems to have left you with the dread that you have.

Most people experience what we call the holiday blues *after* the holidays are over. In your case, it seems your expectations of yourself are so high and your resentment and anxiety have built so much that your blues set in before the holidays have even started. And then, since the holidays are supposedly the "happiest" times, you feel guilty about your response to them, and your feelings of unhappiness are compounded.

Perhaps in the future you can find a way to change things so that you can share in the holiday spirit you have worked so hard to create for others. Examine why you do these things — are you working so hard in an attempt to please others without a thought for yourself? Try getting others to help carry some of the burden you've had over the years with members of your family and take a more relaxed attitude about the gifts you buy and the gatherings you organize.

74

Tell your family and friends how you feel; they may be very surprised to learn that you are not happy with the situation. Too often we think others automatically *know* how we feel — we expect them to read our minds — and when we speak up, we may learn that others don't even want the sacrifices we are making for them.

❦

Celebrating Hanukkah and Keeping the Family Faith

My sixteen-year-old says the stories of Hanukkah are "legends and fairy tales," and he doesn't see any sense in celebrating them. Should I insist that he do so? Are these religious customs as "pointless" as he says they are?

Religious observances do indeed continue to have real value. For many people, they are a way of staying in touch with their past, and with the spiritual and moral values certain traditions represent. Children especially enjoy participating with other members of their family in these cultural and religious celebrations, particularly when they are pleasant and the children are made to feel a part of them. The feeling of family unity that results gives a child a sense of true security, which persists over the years.

It is also true that some people are much more bound by tradition than others. Especially in such families, young people, in their efforts to achieve independence, may show their rebelliousness by refusing to share in religious traditions. In the same way that other young people may question or disparage their family's political views or lifestyle, certain teenagers find fault with their family's religious beliefs, dismissing them as superstition or "legends."

In most cases, these young people return to their family traditions after they've acquired their independence and no longer have to rebel. Their period of questioning in many cases will eventually result in an even greater devotion to their family's faith. They have examined their beliefs and have come to see that they represent deep and abiding spiritual values.

It's important for you to hold your ground and be firm in maintaining these traditions in spite of your son's skepticism. Allow your sixteen-year-old to refrain from participating if he insists; if you try to force him to take part, he will only be more adamant in his stand, and the pleasure of everyone else will be affected. But, whether it "makes sense" to him or not, under no circumstances should you allow him to interfere with what the rest of the family chooses to do.

❦

Anger at Parents' Absence

Our five-year-old is usually sensitive and good-natured. But this evening when we returned from a party with a surprise gift for him, he became very angry. "I don't want it," he yelled. Later, he played happily with the toy, but his initial reaction was very negative, and he has behaved this way on similar occasions. I wonder if he is embarrassed at such emotional moments and doesn't want to be the center of attention — or is it something deeper?

It sounds to me as if his anger about the gift may be anger toward you. Frequently, when parents go away for varying lengths of time, their children resent it and sometimes even feel abandoned by them. This is particularly true if parents leave without any forewarning or adequate preparation. Young children are very dependent upon their parents and resent them for leaving. When they return, it's not uncommon for a child to turn away from the parents and show more interest in whoever cared for him while the parents were gone. Some children will ignore the gifts that the parents bear with them on their return and may show open anger and hostility toward the gift, which is, in a sense, a displacement of their anger toward the parents for having left them in the first place. Needless to say, your child is happy about your return, but he is still angry that you left him. It's not that he doesn't appreciate the gift, it's that he basically prefers you to any object as an exchange. I suggest that you accept his feelings when this occurs and that you be casual in the presentation of any surprise you get him in the future. If he rejects it, simply put it aside and tell him, "I'll leave it here, and whenever you feel ready, it's yours to open and enjoy."

❦

The Child Who Hits His Parents, I

When my two-year-old is angry because I've told him he can't have or do something, he hits me. "Bad Mommy," he'll say, flailing at me again and again. I never quite know how to react to these outbursts. My mother-in-law says I should just spank him. "You can't reason with a two-year-old," she says. Should I hit back? Is a two-year-old capable of understanding what I say to him about this? How can I get it across to him that anger is acceptable but that it shouldn't be vented by hitting people? Is this behavior normal in a two-year-old?

Most two-year-olds have trouble dealing with feelings of anger. It is not uncommon for them to burst into fits of rage and to throw — or even destroy — playthings. Young children have difficulty controlling their emotions and accepting limits; they want what they want when they want it. They are persistent in asserting their independence, and they resist anyone who hinders their efforts. It *is* extremely difficult to reason with children of this age. Although they are certainly people capable of feeling anger, they are not yet intellectually able to "understand" the reasons behind what is happening.

Since two-year-olds tend to imitate their parents, and want to do the things that other children do, they may "hit" because they see their playmates do it. Also, if children observe parents acting out their anger in a physical way, youngsters are likely to take this as an example of how to behave. For this reason, it is absolutely *not* advisable for parents to respond to a child's blows by hitting back. This only reinforces the child's aggressive behavior.

Parents *should* let a child know how they feel about "hitting" by voicing their displeasure in a firm tone of voice and with a stern facial expression. Don't hesitate to stop a child's attack by holding his arms or hands firmly while you let your own feelings be known. Don't be alarmed by your child's outcries against you. Your son has a perfect right and need to express his feelings verbally. In fact, if parents are so punitive that they deny their children the right to express their anger in *any* way, the damming up of this natural feeling can be the beginning of problems that will continue into a child's later life. And it's especially important for children to learn that they can express anger toward loved ones without feeling that it will cause their alienation. By permitting your son to express his feelings verbally, while you restrain and discourage him from responding physically, you are guiding him toward acceptable ways to express his anger.

❦

The Child Who Hits His Parents, II

My six-year-old hits me! Since the age of two, he's done this, and although I've never literally "hit" back, I must admit I'm sorely tempted at times when he's flailing out at me in a fit of temper. How do you handle children who hit their parents?

You have a perfect right to be very angry when your child hits you. In fact, you should have stopped this behavior a long time ago. You simply have to make it absolutely clear that it makes you angry and upset with him. Make your anger clear by your facial expression and tone of voice. When he hits you, grab his hands and restrain him from lashing out at you; but do not hurt him, and restrain him only while he struggles to hit you. Let him know it is all right for him to be angry with you from time to time and that it is fine for him to express his anger verbally — but under no circumstances will you allow him to hit you. Children need to learn to develop internal controls over the enactment of their strongest feelings, and they do this by seeing how their parents handle their own anger. If you strike your child because he hits you, you are indeed condoning such behavior and at the same time showing him that you, too, do not have control over your feelings.

If parents seem to cower under physical attacks by children, or if parents take an indifferent attitude toward their occurrence, it can frighten children and make them anxious about how to deal with their destructive tendencies. Anger and hostility are normal human emotions, but they are ones that need to be controlled, channeled, or directed in some way that is socially acceptable.

It is frequently difficult to teach children some of the more subtle ways of dealing with anger when they themselves are in the midst of their actual rage. It is best to do this when the child has finally calmed down, or at other times when communication between a parent and child is relaxed and going well. You then can be open and direct in explaining how certain things anger people and cause them to flare up, sometimes giving them the impulse to lash out or to break or throw something. Explain further that many people turn their anger into work or redirect it into sports activities or other physical activities. Tell your son that hitting a tennis ball, chopping wood, and jogging are forms of activity that help people relieve the discomfort they feel from angry feelings that have been built up. The most important thing for you to get across to your child is that it is all right to be angry, but it is *not* all right to hit others.

❦

Anger and Hostility in Play-Fantasy

Sometimes my five-year-old and her friends will be playing peacefully with their dolls when suddenly one of them will give her doll a hearty spanking for being "bad." My little boy sometimes does the same thing with his beloved "teddy." It's startling to see this happen in what is otherwise an angelic scene. What is going on when children do this?

Play is one way in which children learn to come to terms with their feelings. It gives them an opportunity to vent their emotions — confusing emotions that they may be frightened of expressing otherwise — by displacing them onto a doll or stuffed animal. It also allows them to act out behavior that they see or sense in their own parents and thus relieve feelings of anxiety that they themselves may have. For instance, children who feel guilty for some transgression may expiate their guilt in play by pretending the doll has been the delinquent. In essence, the child is saying, "It wasn't *me* who did something wrong, it was my doll." By administering the punishment, the child can gain some relief from his or her guilt.

While hostility in play may reflect a child's confusion over expressions of anger, it does not necessarily mean that the child has emotional problems. Playacting is a socially acceptable way for a child to vent anger, guilt, or anxiety. In fact, it is common for psychologists to use play as a diagnostic instrument to gain insight into problems young children may have, particularly if they cannot verbalize their feelings directly. Through play, it's possible to help children work through some of their problems to achieve relief from inner conflicts and tensions. Play is a perfectly healthy outlet for a child's feelings.

❦

Discipline without Spanking

My sister-in-law never strikes her children. In fact, she doesn't discipline them at all, and they're growing up without any real guidelines about what is right and wrong. I think in some people's minds there is confusion between disciplining children and striking them. Does "not hitting" mean you don't discipline children in any way?

Punishing children by physical means does not convince them that something they've done is wrong. Such behavior *does* convince them that you are angry, out of control, unreasonable, and someone to be feared. This can serve to make them feel self-righteous rather than repentant, and the lesson a child comes away with is "next time be careful and don't get caught." In other words, children in such cases learn to control themselves to avoid punishment rather than to deal with the fact that their behavior is not acceptable.

What we want children to develop is a conscience — a humane and compassionate concept of right and wrong — rather than a superficial shrewdness about staying out of trouble. By their observations, children can learn that when people are fair and kind to others and treat them with respect, others are likely to respond in the same way. But if they do things that hurt or annoy people, others in turn will be less friendly and less yielding when it comes to sharing experiences or simply having fun together. But these ideas and attitudes are conveyed by example rather than by physical punishment.

Because they do not involve physical force does not mean that parental guidelines should be any less firm. I strongly believe in discipline and feel that both children and adults require certain guidelines for their behavior. In fact, I'm convinced that people feel *more* comfortable when rules and regulations are clear, well defined, and upheld. Parents should emphasize by their manner and tone of voice that certain behavior is *not* permissible, and that if it continues, certain privileges will be taken away. Parental values and standards of behavior — and the reasons behind them — should be made clear to children, and rules for their enactment should be consistently maintained.

❦

Why Babies Cry

Our new baby is home from the hospital now — and crying constantly! My mother and aunt say the baby's "colicky," but I don't understand what this means. Is he crying because of physical discomfort, or are there emotional reasons for his wailing?

In my experience, babies cry for four basic reasons. One, out of boredom; they need stimulation and attention and need to be held, carried, talked to, and fondled. Two, oftentimes children cry because they are tired and need to be rocked or given some other help in relaxing. Three, many babies cry because of their need for sucking gratification; they generally satisfy this need in the course of the feeding process and in those extra moments of nursing that take place after they have had their fill of food. Four, babies cry because of physical discomfort, because something is too cold or too hot or poking them, or because of some pain they feel inside. Colic is among those physical pains.

When such constant crying continues, it seems as if nothing the parents can do provides relief. This in turn generally makes both mother and father tense, nervous, and frustrated. Often this irritability is communicated back to the child and makes matters even worse. For this reason, many doctors blame parental tension for setting off and prolonging attacks of colic. I disagree. I think colic is caused by real physical pain, which occurs when the baby's formula disagrees with his digestive system. I believe that not all the openings from one part of an infant's digestive system to another are sufficiently wide enough for food to get through easily. Because of this, there can be a buildup of gas and pressure that can cause severe pain. Usually, within a matter of months, when the digestive system has matured, these passageways open sufficiently to allow food to pass through without discomfort, and the attacks of colic subside dramatically.

If your baby seems colicky, discuss with your pediatrician the possibility of changing his formula. Continue to cuddle your baby and offer as much comfort as you possibly can; even though it appears that all your efforts are in vain, an infant still benefits from the closeness and warmth of being held in your arms. In my experience, colicky babies who have been held and cuddled in this way emerge into charming, happy infants as soon as the colic subsides.

Dealing with Crying Babies

I know that you advocate picking up crying babies. But my eighteen-month-old still fusses when he's put down for a nap or in his playpen — and I don't know if it's right for me to run and cuddle him whenever he lets out a peep. How long should a parent cater to a small child's crying and fussing for no apparent reason?

I believe babies always cry for a reason; we just don't always know what that reason is. Very early in life, when they're passive, helpless infants, they can't do much for themselves. They need to have someone who is responsive and who will alleviate the cause of their discomfort. During this infantile stage, if their needs are "catered to," they learn to trust other people and come to see the world as a safe and satisfying place. But the child who is left to cry it out has virtually no alternative but to find solace by tuning out the world and going off to sleep. If this becomes a characteristic pattern for dealing with the stresses of infancy, it later on might continue to be the first line of defense in dealing with any kind of stress. I'm convinced that severely withdrawn children and adults, as well as those people who go off to sleep rather than face problems and solve them, come to think early in infancy that no one in their lives is responsive enough to help them cope.

When a child gets to be ten or eleven months of age, however, and wakes up at night, I don't suggest that you rush to pick him or her up immediately. I do feel, though, that you should try to comfort your child while he's still in his crib by patting his back, caressing him a little, and letting him know you are there and he is not abandoned. If you find that your baby simply wants to socialize in the middle of the night, I don't suggest that you encourage it. Instead, put your baby back down in his crib and try to comfort him. If he continues to get up, crying to have you play with him, put him down each time

in a firm yet patient and gentle manner. Eventuallv he will get
the message that you are there but that you will not pick him
up and play at that hour of the night. You may have to put him
down as many as thirty or forty times to convince him of this,
but.at least you are being consistent in discouraging him while
staying with him for support.

❦

Starting Discipline

*My son is almost seven months old, and I have been trying to
stop him from touching things on my coffee table and shelves,
but he doesn't seem to understand. Some people say I shouldn't
curtail his activity because he needs to feel these things; others
say stop him now or he'll get worse and be into everything; and
still others say to wait to discipline him about this until he's
two years old. Can you tell me at what age I should teach him
he can't touch everything he wants to?*

The age you begin to set such guidelines is determined more
by your child's capabilities than by his chronological age. When
a child begins reaching for things and is able to grasp them and
pull them toward himself, this is the time you have to assist
him in knowing what is permissible behavior and what is not.
By permitting him to touch many things but not all things,
you're still giving him the opportunity of learning how various
textures and shapes feel.

I would like to say that I don't believe in removing everything
from the coffee table or rearranging your surroundings so that
nothing is within a toddler's reach; this doesn't solve the problem, it simply avoids the issue. I would suggest that you take
away especially fragile things or valuable things that may easily

be destroyed by your child and then set conditions as to the other possessions that he *can* and *cannot* touch. Most children at an age when they can reach out and grab things are very curious about all kinds of things. As long as you are not so restrictive that your child is discouraged from exploration gen- erally, you will not be limiting his sense of freedom. In fact, you will be defining certain boundaries in which he must learn to function in order to live successfully with others. This is an im- portant lesson to learn, and since children want and need dis- cipline, they will approach your lessons as they approach a game. Show your dissatisfaction when a child touches or grabs something that is unacceptable. Be firm and and say no em- phatically, but do not overreact in such a way that it will be overwhelming and upsetting to your child. As soon as children realize that certain objects are forbidden, you can be sure they will experiment with you: They will use their other hand to find whether it's the left or right hand, or *both* hands, that triggers your reaction. If you are consistent in your responses and patient enough to allow your child to test out all your possible reactions, your child will eventually learn the "rules" that are appropriate in this situation. Prepare yourself for the fact that he may test you from time to time by doing what he now knows is forbidden — and each time he will probably smile as he does it. While this may make you feel as if he's out to get you, he's not. He simply wants to reaffirm his understanding of what the rules are. It's all somewhat like a game to a child, and gives him a feeling that you really care sufficiently about him to react to what he does, and to establish rules for his behavior.

❦

Being Nervous with a Newborn

I'm the mother of a newborn baby, my first. I'm terribly nervous about handling him, and my husband keeps telling me that I'll transmit my nervousness to the baby. Can this happen? Or am I just being neurotic?

It's perfectly normal for new parents, both mothers and fathers, to be nervous about their newborn babies. In fact, most parents do become anxious when they hear their baby cry. Not only is this normal, but I think it's good! Your anxiety leads you to find out what's wrong so that you can alleviate your baby's discomfort or boredom so that he or she will be happy again. In fact, the mothers of all young mammals have a similar protective instinct and are not only anxious but intensely protective. Everyone knows that touching a baby bear cub that has wandered off from the mother is a very dangerous thing indeed. The bear mother's instinct is to "annihilate" you, no matter how tender and nice you're being to her offspring. It would do you no good to shout at a charging, enraged mother bear that she's overprotective or neurotic.

You can be sure that your initial nervousness about handling your baby will subside as you become more familiar with your new role. At first, mothers are fearful that a baby is so delicate that something harmful will occur if an infant's head is not always supported, or if an arm or leg is accidentally twisted. Remember, though, there's a great deal of squeezing, pushing, and tugging during birth itself, and your baby's hardiness was sufficient to withstand any substantial injury at that time.

As your husband suggests, a parent's anxiousness *can* be communicated to the baby. A nervous mother will handle a baby in a more abrupt manner, and this certainly gets through to the child. Once again, though, infants are very hardy. And while a relaxed manner is best, a normal amount of natural concern is nothing that should affect your baby adversely.

I would like to add that simply pointing out your nervousness does no good. It may, in fact, simply intensify it. It would be far better if your husband, recognizing your fears, would offer you support and reassurance as well as help in dealing with the many new demands that can be at times an overwhelming burden.

❧

The Clinging Child

I'm the mother of an eleven-month-old son. He's our only child, and he's a very lovable baby — but that's part of the trouble. He wants to be held or played with all day long, and there's not one minute I have to myself. When I try to do some housework, he's at my feet, crying and pulling at my leg. If I put him in his playpen, he screams the whole time. I hope you can give me some advice because I'm getting to be a nervous wreck.

This is not at all an uncommon problem. In fact, it's one I discuss with young people who may one day become parents, in an effort to give them a realistic picture of what having a baby is really like, and what the commitment of parenthood actually means. I am sure this isn't the least bit comforting to you at this point, but I simply want to point out that it is a normal and common problem — and believe me, it will not go on indefinitely.

In all likelihood the reason your baby *is* very lovable is because you have been responsive to him and have held him and played with him for long periods of time. But now, to give you some relief, I suggest that you ask or employ someone who likes babies and enjoys playing with them to come and help you for a few hours a day or a few times a week. Don't turn your child over to this person abruptly, but have the newcomer spend time with both you and your baby during the first few visits. Eventually, as the new relationship grows, you will find it easier to leave your child with his new companion, leaving you more free time for your work and interests.

It's as important for your child to learn to respond to other people as it is for you to have some relief from the pressures of being a parent. However, it's also important to do this in a way that doesn't create an intense anxiety in your child. Your baby wants *you* because he trusts you and finds your presence satisfying. Now it's time to help him understand that you will always be close by if he needs you but that there are other people in this world who are also responsive and loving.

❦

Family Bonding

My daughter and her husband recently had a baby — and almost immediately started taking the infant with them on errands, picnics, and a variety of other activities. The other night they even took him to a bowling alley! I think such carrying on is certainly too rough for a delicate infant and that they should be more careful. What do you think?

I think it's marvelous when people take their babies with them wherever they go. Not only does it strengthen their family bond, but it provides the baby with a feeling of security and trust in the parents. Moreover, babies who are cared for in this way learn to adapt more easily to variations in sights and sounds and are not easily distressed by a change in routine. They learn to sleep through anything, eat different kinds of food, and are less likely to become distressed by strangers and new experiences.

If things get to be too much for their baby, you can be sure they'll know about it. The baby's cry is a signal of distress, and it unquestionably will be heard if things get rough. By the same token, that look of contentment, broken periodically by giggles and smiles, reflects happiness. Babies have a way of letting their parents know how they feel, and these feelings should always be acknowledged and respected.

❦

Being Close to Your Newborn

A friend recently mentioned that, after the birth of her baby, she hadn't actually held her infant until "the next day or so." I was alarmed to hear this. I hope to become pregnant soon, and I think it's important to hold a newborn as soon as possible. Don't you agree?

I'm absolutely convinced that the period immediately following birth is critical in the establishment of strong ties between parent and child. I agree that you should make every effort possible in advance of the birth to make sure you will be allowed immediate and free contact with your newborn baby. In fact, in selecting your physician in the first place, you should find out what hospital he or she is affiliated with and then check its procedures in these matters.

I was happy to learn that the American Medical Association issued a statement urging all hospitals to examine their existing procedures and, taking into consideration the research findings on the subject of the bonding process between mothers and newborn infants, revise their regulations to make childbirth the most rewarding experience possible for parents and infant.

❦

Teenager Always Late

Our teenager is always late! When she makes a date to meet us — or any of her friends, for that matter — she may keep us waiting for a half hour or longer. All of us are getting terribly irritated with her. How should we handle her chronic lateness?

There is no reason for you to put up with your daughter's behavior. By tolerating her constant lateness and allowing her to make excuses, you are simply condoning her actions. No matter how many explanations she gives, the simple fact is that her pattern of lateness causes aggravation and inconvenience for those waiting.

As long as your daughter gets away with being late, and without "punishments," she will disregard the rules — and she will never learn a pattern of behavior that will be constructive to her throughout her lifetime. Therefore, if she does not arrive on time for certain activities, she should simply be excluded. If she is late coming home when the family is going to a movie, go without her. If she is continually late for meals, don't cater to her by waiting or reheating food for her, but let her eat leftovers. If her friends also let her know that they will wait for her a short time but no longer — and will simply go on without her if she is not there — her lateness should soon become inconvenient for *her* rather than for *others*. Ultimately she will learn a lesson that should make the rest of her life happier and easier.

❦

Teenager and Privacy

My fourteen-year-old daughter makes a big production of writing in her diary and announcing how "private" it all is — and then leaves it around in plain sight on the kitchen counter or coffee table. The other day, as I was dusting, I couldn't help it — I opened her diary and saw an account of how she and her friends were smoking and drinking at a recent party, things that she's expressly forbidden to do. Now my problem is how to talk to her about this without revealing my source. How can I do this? And don't you think if she left the diary prominently exposed like this, she wanted me to read it?

Being a parent can certainly be exasperating; and a situation such as this certainly proves it. It *is* fair to assume that her leaving her diary sitting around is for the purpose of having you read it. But this doesn't mean you should. Telling you it's "private" and practically putting it under your nose is her way of testing your actual respect for her privacy. In one way, she's asking you to violate her rights by tempting you with information about smoking and drinking — and she can then be "devastated" and filled with moral indignation if and when you talk to her about this.

I believe you will teach her a lesson by not rising to the bait and revealing what you know. Instead, point out that she is *not* to leave her diary around and unattended. Tell her that if she does, you will consider it a "public document" and will take the liberty of reading it. Emphasize the fact that it's her responsibility to guard the contents of something that she is theoretically so sensitive about. Once you've pointed this out to her, you are in a far better position to eventually cope with the rules that she is breaking — at another time and under other circumstances (after all, the news of what she is doing is bound to "slip out" somehow in another way). If you let her know about reading the diary now, you'll be playing into her hands and giving her justification for never trusting you again.

Fear of Growing Up

I'm a twelve-year-old girl who's scared of growing up. My friend wants to do it! She talks about wearing makeup and going out on dates and to dances and things like that — stuff that really makes me feel funny. Are all kids scared of growing up? Or is there something wrong with me?

Not only is there nothing wrong with you for feeling the way you do, but I admire you for being concerned enough and strong enough to ask for help.

Many young people have fears that you have. Life is, in a sense, a series of changes in our feelings, desires, and needs. As we pass through various stages of life, these changes can cause confusion and uncertainty, and the problems they present can appear insurmountable; most of this works out in time, and new feelings become more comfortable as we develop as individuals.

Right now, at your particular age, there can be great differences, both physically and mentally, among young people. Your friend who talks about dates and dances may indeed be as uneasy about the future as you are, and her way of dealing with her fears may be to talk confidently about "growing up" in order to convince herself that everything will be all right in the changing years ahead. Everyone handles fears and worries in different ways, and each person grows at a different pace. As time passes, things that now seem strange and frightening to you will one day become a natural and exciting new part of your life.

❦

Teenagers and Dolls

Although my daughter is nearly thirteen and in junior high school, she still plays with her dolls and stuffed animals. Her other friends all seem to be interested in dances, rock music, and boys. I wonder if I should be worried about my daughter's development. Should I pressure her to give up her toys for more normal teenage activities?

Your daughter is on the borderline between childhood and adolescence, at a time of life when social maturity varies from child to child. But, in general, when a youngster does take that step into a more "grownup" life, it is rather dramatic, and many parents are frequently shocked at its abruptness. They can hardly believe that their "sweet little girl" has emerged into an independent peer-oriented admirer of dancing, music, and the opposite sex (especially when it seems that only the day before, her reaction to boys was *"yeck"*).

I don't think you should be worried about your daughter's development, nor do I think you should pressure her to make any changes before she is ready. Some children cling to their childhood interests longer than others. If, however, an inordinate interest in playing with dolls continues well beyond the time she shows pubescent physical development, you might then consider the possibility of an underlying emotional problem and seek competent psychological help for her if it seems necessary.

❦

Teenagers and Religious Rebellion

Ever since our children were very small, our family has always attended religious services together. But now our sixteen-year-old son has begun to balk at going along — he says he doesn't "believe that stuff" any more. My husband and I are very upset about this, and the issue has begun to cause great tension. My husband and I have strong religious convictions that we feel should be passed on to our children, but what do you do when the children resist?

The more you try to force your son, the more he will balk at attending religious services. He is going through a stage in his development when he is trying to assert himself, to show his independence and establish his individuality. For many young people in our culture, it is very difficult to achieve self-reliance without rebelling against the very people on whom they have been dependent. Frequently they reject their parents' beliefs simply in order to assert themselves.

Show the same respect for his feelings that you want him to show for yours. Let him know how strongly you feel about this, but at the same time let him know that you have no intention of forcing him to accept your beliefs. If you make every effort to understand the struggle he is going through, and if you allow him to work things out in his own way, you leave open the option for him to join you in your religious beliefs and observances at another time. Also, if young people feel a real emotional security throughout their family life, there is a great likelihood that they will remain members of that family unit in spite of a divergence in religious views. They will return to share in family festivities, many of which center around religious holidays.

❦

Teenage Socializing

My teenage daughter had been spending a lot of time with one of the "popular" boys in her high school. Then, without explanation, he stopped seeing her and started spending all his time with another girl. When I asked her about it, she said, "Oh, who cares?" But she's been very listless and depressed since the break-up, and her studies and activities don't seem to interest her any more. What's happening? Is there a way I can help her get over this disappointment?

In all likelihood, your daughter's superficial attitude of nonchalance is a defensive reaction that psychologists call "denial"; it's a way of avoiding a painful situation by pretending — most of all to oneself — that it didn't happen. But it is normal for people to feel angry or sad about the loss of someone who was important to them. And whatever the disappointment or upset, people must experience their feelings of frustration, anger, and sadness before they can move on to other things. To deny an experience from the start and pretend it didn't matter can only cause a buildup of psychological problems and even physical symptoms.

It takes a great deal of psychological energy for a person to repress his or her real feelings. Your daughter's efforts to smother her pain and anger require so much energy that she is left feeling listless, tired, and depressed. This also weakens her motivation to do other things and leaves her more vulnerable to illness.

If your daughter would express her rage and indignation, she would be greatly relieved. You can help her do this by encouraging her to talk about and deal with her real feelings, as difficult as it may be. Do not tell her she "shouldn't feel that way" or should "snap out of it because things aren't so bad." This only reinforces her attitude of denial and makes it seem as though you are disinterested in her problems and would rather deal

96

with things superficially instead of working to help her seek out the truth.

The best way to help people who are feeling this kind of depression is to provide them with opportunities to express their feelings, and to respond to them with compassion and understanding when they do.

❦

Teenage Childish Behavior

My daughter is fourteen, but I still often discover her in her room playing with her dolls and stuffed animals, or moving figures and furniture around in her dollhouse. How long do young girls continue to do this? One day when I asked her what she was doing, her eyes filled up with tears and she refused to talk about it. Is this something I should worry about?

It's always important to remember that every child is different and that each one matures at a different rate. Many teenagers remain attached to some of their childhood toys, and keep stuffed animals in their rooms long after childhood. It is unusual, however, for a fourteen-year-old to actually "play" in a dollhouse, particularly if this is one of her primary activities. But what concerns me the most about your daughter is her reaction to your question about what she was doing. Her tearfulness and refusal to talk about her feelings indicate that there are pent-up emotions associated with her play activity. There is a possibility that your daughter is emotionally blocked or unable to resolve her concerns and should receive professional psychological counseling to help her work through whatever upsetting emotions she may have.

Children frequently act out their innermost feelings in fantasy and play, and sometimes learn to deal with their emotions more effectively by doing so. A child's need to engage over and over again in a given activity, such as acting out a certain family drama with dollhouse figures, may mean that she is trying desperately to resolve a conflict in her life.

The medium of play is frequently used by child psychologists and psychiatrists to help their young patients come to terms with their feelings. Children who have difficulty verbalizing their emotions directly can do so more comfortably by attributing their confused feelings and unacceptable impulses to doll-like figures, thus giving a therapist insight into what is bothering the child. A child such as your daughter sounds like an excellent candidate for psychotherapy because of the ease with which she can engage in fantasy play, as well as because of the discomfort she must be experiencing as a result of her pent-up feelings. The more uncomfortable a person feels, the more motivated he or she is to accept help for troubling problems.

❦

Imaginary Playmates

My five-year-old boy blames his imaginary friend "George" for a lot of things that he does himself. When something is spilled or torn or broken, he says that "George did it." What's going on when a child insists that an imaginary person is responsible for mischief and wrongdoing? Can make-believe playmates be emotionally harmful for a child?

The presence of a make-believe playmate is not emotionally harmful as long as your child is aware that it *is* make-believe — and that you know this, too. It is important for children to be able to make the distinction between what is real and what is pretend. Some parents are afraid that they will rob a child of the pleasure of play by making this clear, but their fears are unfounded. Children can relate quite vividly and emotionally to make-believe events, and this gives them great latitude for the expression of their ideas and feelings.

Children sometimes try to resolve the real problems of their lives through their play, and it sounds to me as if your five-year-old child is trying to do just that. By attributing his own misbehavior to George, your son has found a great way to engage in "unacceptable" activities and at the same time live a life free of guilt. Needless to say, it's unwise to allow children to absolve themselves of their misdeeds without some feelings of remorse or punishment. Let your son know that George is certainly welcome in your house, but that your son is the one responsible for all the things that his imaginary playmate does and that he will have to pay the consequences of George's wrongdoings. If you handle the situation in this way, I predict that the imaginary George will shape up — or else your son will send him on his way as easily as he conjured him up in the first place.

❧

Hero Worship

My ten-year-old daughter's idol is Dorothy Hamill, and she talks about how she is going to be "just like her and win medals at the Olympics." But it's clear that she doesn't have the talent to become a champion (her skating teacher agrees with me about this). Is it good for children to have "idols" such as this, or is my daughter just being set up for disappointment later on?

The people that the majority of children "worship" or admire represent values and characteristics that are socially valuable and beneficial and that bring others satisfaction and pleasure. When children pick someone to idolize, they too want the recognition and the sense of pride and achievement that these heroes have.

Under no circumstances belittle your child's intense desires to emulate a figure of strength or talent — but you might make it clear that no one will ever be Dorothy Hamill but Dorothy Hamill herself. Support your daughter in her desire to do an outstanding job. Let her know that you admire her effort and diligence; tell her that while she *may* not achieve her goals, you will always admire her for pursuing them and doing the best job she could. At the same time, do not encourage her to achieve something that far exceeds her ability; even as you support her efforts and her diligence, help her to be realistic in evaluating her own abilities and setting her own goals. I believe that children — and everyone else, for that matter — should compete not with others but with themselves, continually striving to improve their own skills

❦

Teenage Rebellion

All of a sudden my sweet-natured teenager is a stranger! She's irritable and demanding about everything — and whatever I want her to do, she does the opposite. Would you say something comforting, please, about adolescent rebellion? When does it begin and end! Why does it happen? Is this a normal stage of development all kids go through, and why?

Adolescent rebellion does not exist in all societies or cultures throughout the world. Scientists such as Margaret Mead who studied adolescence in different cultures seemed to agree that in cultures where teenagers could make the transition from childhood to adulthood easily and quickly, with acceptance and support from the adult members of that community, rebelliousness either did *not* occur or was minimal. The "rites of passage" or other rituals that young people go through in some primitive societies help make that transition cleanly and quickly, thus avoiding the long period of parental dependency that teenagers in our culture experience.

As I have counseled many parents and teenagers over the years, I've come to the conclusion that teenagers are *not* as rebellious as many people think. Unquestionably we see evidence of rebelliousness during teenage years, but I believe this is caused to a great extent by the inability of parents and other adult authorities in our society to accept what is part of the normal development that all young people go through as they grow to maturity. Rebelliousness, in my mind, results when adults fail to adapt themselves to this rapid growth. When young people become physically larger in size and begin to mature sexually, they understandably want to act in more of the ways that our culture considers "adult." Parents who are reluctant to see their "babies" grow up, frequently — consciously or unconsciously — attempt to hold them back. This is frustrating, embarrassing, and painful to the young people involved.

If we insist that adolescents follow our dictates and accept our values, we can be sure that they will rebel against us. In fact, this is true not only for adolescents but in any other situation in life where people attempt to exercise power over others. When children are younger, parents are indeed larger, stronger, and in a position to control the behavior of their children; but as children grow to adolescence, parents no longer have the same power.

Your "sweet-natured" teenager has not become a stranger. She's simply growing up, and this means that you must change your perceptions of her and learn to give her more freedom and independence so that she can develop her own personal skills for being independent and responsible. Bear in mind that she will make mistakes, will demand to do things her own way, and may instantly shift her opinions from one extreme to another as part of this process.

At these times many parents become anxious that their teenagers might be hurt, and so they try to tell them what to do instead of allowing them to work things out for themselves. That is why you as a parent must allow your child to take the risks necessary for personal growth. If you make yourself available to your daughter, and express your sincere love and desire to help if she gets into trouble, she will probably turn to you if any misfortune occurs. But some parents say, in effect, "Do it my way — or don't come running to me if you need help." An ultimatum of this sort may drive your teenager away from you and cause her to turn to a peer group for the emotional support that you've withdrawn. During this time parents need, in a sense, to treat their teenagers both as responsible, functioning adults and as little children who may run to them for help during periods of despair.

Several years ago, while returning from my summer vacation in Maine, my son, Eric, who was fourteen at the time, was shopping for shoes. I pointed to some loafers and asked what he thought about them. His response was *"Yech!"* There was no discussion between us; I simply moved on and suggested he look for something he liked. After driving another twenty minutes, we stopped at a big shoe outlet and he said, "Dad! *These* are the ones I want." They were exactly the same shoes we had seen twenty minutes before. I said, "Fine, let's get them." I then added, "You know, Eric, I can understand why you like these shoes and hated the ones you saw before." The reason he liked these and not the others was simply because he was now twenty minutes older than he was before. There were no arguments, there was no rebelliousness, but there was understanding of his need to assert himself and to do things in his own way.

❧

Talking to Teenagers

My thirteen-year-old just mutters or scowls — she won't speak up about what's on her mind. It frustrates me terriby to have our communication so cut off in this way. How can I get her to open up to me?

She may have trouble speaking with you if you in some way have played a role in causing the confusion she feels. On the other hand, she may feel misunderstood by you if you have in any way demeaned her or her ideas. I don't think you should feel unloved or that your opinions are unimportant.

Let your daughter know that you understand that she must be troubled by something. Don't probe or pressure her — that will be sure to cause her to balk — but simply let her know that you're available to listen if there is something on her mind and that you would like to help her become happier. Don't try to be a pal or buddy or in any way talk the language of teenagers — that is sure to be a "turn-off."

Don't hesitate to let your daughter know that you, too, in your life have had moments when you were angry, frustrated, and confused. Tell her that you're sure that when the time comes and she feels like discussing anything, you will be there to offer whatever help you can. If her agitation grows and is accompanied by tearfulness, depression, and even further withdrawal, then I feel you should seek professional help and urge her to speak with someone who is trained to help people with their discomfort.

❦

Parental Teasing

My husband teases our four-year-old, telling her she's "chubby as a watermelon" and calling her "potato face" and "chipmunk cheeks," and things like that. I imagine she must be hurt by his remarks, but when I tell him so, he says I'm being silly. Is a young child sophisticated enough to realize that he's only joking? Aren't his comments having a detrimental effect on her? Or am I just getting upset over nothing?

Some people do express their affection in a somewhat teasing or joking manner, and your husband's remarks are apparently made in that spirit. Most children can sense when their parents mean to express affection in this way, and they are generally not upset or hurt by those remarks unless they touch on a particularly embarrassing area. A child concerned about being overweight, for instance, would hardly appreciate being called "fatty," no matter how fondly! In that case, such a "joke" is downright hostile.

But children vary in their sensitivity to joking remarks, just as they vary in all other respects. And parents are generally sufficiently tuned in to their children's reactions to know whether a child is demoralized or hurt. But if there is any question in your mind as to how your child is taking this, how she feels about being called these names, explain that her father loves her and says these things as a joke, and that he has no intention of hurting her. Tell her if she prefers not to be teased in this way, you will make sure it stops. And at that point, instead of *imagining* how your daughter feels, you will have something concrete to deal with when you discuss this with your husband.

❧

Teasing the Overweight Child

Our nine-year-old is becoming increasingly overweight. She snacks constantly, and the teasing of her brothers and sisters about how "tubby" she's getting doesn't seem to affect her at all. And since her siblings are able to eat whatever they want without gaining a pound, it seems cruel to single one child out and refuse her dessert when the rest of us are enjoying cakes and ice cream. My husband says not to worry, that she'll "grow out" of her pudginess. Is he right, or is it important to check these eating habits now? And if it is, isn't it psychologically damaging to be deprived, or nagged at, while others are enjoying sweets?

Some problems subside spontaneously with time, while others become more complicated unless you intervene early. True, your daughter might outgrow her pudginess, but I think it's too risky to take that chance. Unquestionably, you should consult your pediatrician and see just how your daughter is progressing physically. You might find that in spite of what appears as a weight gain to you, she is showing normal growth and development. If, however, she really is becoming heavier day by day, as you think, it would certainly be best to work out a sensible eating schedule that will provide her with low-calorie foods she likes. Nagging her serves no purpose whatsoever, and ridiculing her can lead to feelings of rejection. The more rejected and isolated she becomes, the less she will feel like an accepted member of the family, and this can only compound her problem.

Of course, it would be cruel to deprive your daughter of cakes and ice cream while her siblings are allowed to eat to their hearts' content. Ideally, you should try to keep tempting foods out of her sight. This can best be done by changing the entire family's diet. It is possible to plan meals for your whole family that will be tasty yet low in calories. Children who enjoy sweets can learn to be satisfied with fruit especially if you keep a supply of it in the house instead of cookies and snacks. It is important, however, to make it clear that you are modifying these eating habits for the entire family's benefit, as a means of preventing health problems for everyone in the future. This will protect your daughter from the rejection of her brothers and sisters, who may blame her for these changes.

Policing your daughter's eating habits when she is away from home is difficult. There is little you can do to prevent her from eating candies at school or in friends' homes. Hopefully, once your new family diet has helped her develop tastes for nutritionally healthy food, those tastes will accompany her everywhere. As your daughter loses weight, the taunting by classmates and siblings, unquestionably a great source of unhappiness for the overweight child, will subside, and will free her from such teasing.

❦

Children's Racial Remarks

My four-year-old son goes to a nursery school in the city where we live. The other day, while he was playing, he came out with a racial epithet that shocked me — he's certainly never heard it in our house. I told him in a horrified voice that he must never ever say such a thing, then later in the afternoon I heard him use it again. I'm dreadfully upset that my child may be turning into a little bigot. How should I deal with the situation? Am I overreacting to its importance?

Your concern about this is commendable, and your reaction is completely understandable. Children are highly impressionable about what they see and hear and frequently imitate the behavior and remarks of their parents and peers.

It was appropriate to let him know that you were shocked and horrified, but you must also discuss this matter with him in more detail. However, if he fears you will punish him, reject him, or cause trouble for him, he will be reluctant to tell you where he's heard these remarks and who says them. Therefore, let him know you're not angry with him, but make it clear that such remarks show a lack of respect and can cause very real hurt to the people to whom they refer. Explain that people who use such demeaning expressions are weak and frightened inside themselves — they are not people who are friendly, sure of themselves, and well liked.

While it may be difficult to get these ideas across to a four-year-old, I'm sure you know your child well enough to know how best to convey your concern. It is always better to let a child know the literal consequences of his remarks and behavior rather than take a strictly prohibitive attitude about them. If you simply "forbid" your child to say such things, your prohibitions can work only while you're present to hear him. Instead, your child needs help in developing an attitude of his own about unacceptable behavior. Tell him that such remarks are unjust and offensive and in the long run will cause him to lose friends. Explain that they are shocking to some people, even though others might consider them funny. If he sees the possibility of social rejection as a consequence of his acts, it will serve to modify his language far more than an unexplained prohibition for using these remarks.

If you find that certain of his friends in particular use these expressions, you might contact the parents of these children and discuss the matter with them in a friendly and open-minded way. While they may be hostile to you and take your inquiry as a personal affront, it is still your responsibility to protect the integrity of other human beings in this way. On the other hand, they may be very appreciative of the fact that you brought this to their attention so that they, too, can do something about it.

I think you should also take this opportunity to speak to

school authorities to find out if they have observed children in your son's class using these expressions. This will give you a chance to suggest that the nursery school teacher select some children's books to read to her class that express friendship and respect for people of all backgrounds, beliefs, and colors.

❧

Naming Your Child

I'll be having a baby — our first — in a few months. If it's a boy, my husband feels strongly that we should name him Elmer for his father and grandfather — "to carry on a proud family tradition." I think it's unfair to burden a child with a name that his peers are likely to make fun of as he's growing up. Does an unusual name affect a child?

Parents can sometimes go too far in giving children unusual names that leave them highly vulnerable to the teasing of other children. Nevertheless, there is no way you can avoid picking a name that will be entirely free of such a possibility. When children are in the mood, they can change even the simplest name into a rhyme or joke for their amusement. More often than not, it's the relationship children have with one another that perpetuates the teasing and not the name itself.

However, I've known some children who have been deeply embarrassed by the name they have been given and have felt resentful toward their parents because of it. In such cases, sensitive parents manage to recognize the child's reactions and allow him to adopt a different name or nickname that he can tell his playmates. Generally, children understand a family's desire to maintain a family tradition — as long as they still are allowed to adapt its use to their own individuality. I suggest that a child be given a middle name — even two or three names — among which is the "proud family" one. Then, as the child gets older, he can pick the one most fitting to his desires, while still officially maintaining the name that assures the continuity of family tradition.

❦

Calling Parents by First Names

Some "modern" young children in our neighborhood call their parents by their first names. Do you think it's a good or a bad idea to have your child call you "Dorothy and Eddie" instead of "Mommy and Daddy"? These same parents tell my children, who are ages five through thirteen, to call them by their first names also, and I object to this. Am I being rigid and old-fashioned?

The emotional benefit children gain in their relationships with adults is in no way related to the way in which they address them. Explain to your children that the words we use in greeting people are determined largely by social custom and that respecting the rights and dignity of others is far more important than any titles. Nevertheless, children and adults should respect the wishes of one another in matters both large and small, and if you as parents want to be addressed as mother and father (or Mr. and Mrs. by other children), by all means say so. By the same token, if your children prefer to be called by a nickname or a middle name, you should respect their wishes. And if your children's friends' parents prefer to be addressed by their first names, I see nothing wrong with this.

On the other hand, insisting that a child use first names for adults when he feels awkward about doing so can be wrong.

For some children, "Mommy" and "Daddy" are important words that give them security and support, and "sophisticated" parents should be careful not to deprive their children of these emotionally charged words that can symbolize so much to them.

Basically, my children address adults as Mr. and Mrs. until the adults themselves give permission for their first names to be used. To me, this is the best approach — allowing adults and children alike to become familiar in a framework of respect and courtesy.

❧

"Me First" — the Stubborn Child

Whenever my six-year-old son and four-year-old daughter play a game together, the older child insists on winning, or on playing the games according to rules he sets. He must be the first in everything — going upstairs, having his choice of hamburgers or toys, ordering the first ice-cream cone. Our youngest child doesn't seem to mind as yet, but we don't like this overly dominant attitude in our son. What can we do to curtail it without making him even more stubborn?

It sounds as if your six-year-old doesn't feel secure unless he is first, or, in a sense, the "only one." Being the winner, in his mind, may be the equivalent of being the only child. Remember, he *was* the only one until he was two years of age. When his sister was born, he may have developed doubts about his position in the family, which caused him to need constant reassurance that he is accepted. His greatest feeling of emotional security may have been when he was the only child. In his attempt to recapture that feeling, he fights to be first in everything.

In my experience, this kind of struggle occurs much more often, and with greater intensity, when children are between two and two and a half years apart in age. At two, children are somewhat crude in the expression of their feelings and require substantially more parental time and attention than they do when they are perhaps three years of age or older. It seems evident to me that your six-year-old's competitive spirit has been "fueled" by the two-year age difference between himself and his sister.

Your son is not being as dominant as he is anxious. His anxiety seems to be based on his fear of losing parental love and affection. If you give him more love and affection, as well as your undivided attention, you may find that his competitiveness will subside spontaneously. It would help matters if you explained to him, during those times when communication between you is best, that you love him very much and that your love is undiminished even when he doesn't win games and comes in second, third, or even last. Try to get across the idea that winning or being first has nothing whatsoever to do with your love and acceptance of him.

It would also be helpful if, when he loses a game, or is prevented from being first in ordering his ice-cream cone or hamburger, that you help him cope with his anxiety by showing him, at that very moment, that you love him. It doesn't have to be with words — in fact, it's better communicating with a hug, a reassuring look, or even a kiss. Finally, without being harsh, you can set certain ground rules about going upstairs, or placing food orders, that serve to minimize the number of situations where his drive to be first will occur.

❧

Preparing for the New Baby

I'm pregnant, and within the last few weeks we've told our three-year-old son that another baby will soon arrive in our family. We were as straightforward as possible about this, and have included our son in all the preparations for the newcomer, such as fixing the baby's room. Recently, however, he has taken to wetting his bed every night. What is going on? How should we handle it?

It is very common for young children to regress into this kind of behavior in anticipation of a new sibling. With some children, the reaction comes *after* the birth of the baby, while others react before the baby's actual appearance. Your three-year-old is not at all sure that he likes the change about to take place in his family. From his point of view, this is a great deal of fuss and bother for a tiny baby that no one even knows yet! He is also wondering, "Why do you need a new baby, anyway? Why am *I* not good enough for you?" At the same time, he probably shares some of your enthusiasm and pleasant anticipation. What it all boils down to is a great deal of ambivalence on his part, not unlike some of the ambivalence you yourself must have felt during your pregnancy. Part of him wants to help in the preparations for the new child, but part of him is saying, "*I* want to be that baby everyone is getting excited about." This message comes through in regressive or infantile behavior, such as bedwetting. In a sense, it forces you to take care of him in somewhat the same way you will be caring for that new, unfamiliar brother or sister he is not so sure he wants.

The best way for you to handle the situation is in a low-key, matter-of-fact manner. Don't embarrass or punish your son because of his bedwetting. Tell him that you know he is probably a little nervous about the new baby, but assure him that you love him and will continue to do so, no matter what. Explain that no two children are alike, and even though you will love the new baby and will have to devote time to caring for it, this will in no way change your feelings for him. Give him a little extra love and attention — but don't be nervous as you do so, or behave as if you are doing the wrong thing by having a baby. If his bedwetting doesn't stop even with this extra attention and understanding on your part, it will after the baby is born, and your son realizes that your love for him is unaffected by the newcomer.

❦

Sibling Jealousy

Our five-year-old daughter is very jealous of our four-year-old son and can be very mean to him at times. If he falls down or pinches a finger, she will say, "Oh, goodie!" and when he tries to open the refrigerator to get an apple, she holds the door so he can't get in. These actions are really getting worse, and I don't know what to do. Our boy is very easygoing and is never mean to her. Why might she be doing this? What should we do?

In all likelihood she is doing this because she still feels resentful of his having taken away much of the undivided time and attention she received until he was born. When her brother came along, your daughter was still very young and not capable of understanding the concept of sharing. At that time she was probably still in diapers, still nursing or feeding from a bottle, and very much in need of the kind of personalized care that a dependent one-year-old needs. Had your children been at least three years apart, you could have provided her with the kind of undivided care she needed for that period of her life, until she had grown to understand the idea of sharing. Children under three are rather crude in the expression of their feelings and need a great deal of one-to-one contact with an adult; in fact, they are virtually incapable of engaging in sustained play with another child before this time. It's almost as if the crude feelings your daughter had when she was one year of age were intensified and have persisted until now. She feels her brother is a threat to her and may cause her to lose what she holds dear.

This kind of resentment and jealousy also may result when parents compare siblings to each other. If on occasion you have said to your daughter, "Look how well your little brother behaves — why can't you do the same?" her resentment will only get worse. This sets her baby brother up as a model for acceptable behavior and implies that her brother is more desirable than she is. Episodes or casual remarks like this often occur without much thought on the part of a parent, and they can intensify jealousy and rivalry to a high pitch.

Your daughter is now at an age when you can better reason with her. Let her know, not only with words but with actions, that even though she seems to be very annoyed with her brother, you love her very much. At the same time, make a special effort to take an interest in the things that give her a feeling of recognition and pride. Show her that you are proud of her accomplishments and are available to help her cope with any of the problems that arise in her everyday life. Once you establish this pattern of interest and support, you are in a better position to deal firmly with her hostility. Let her know clearly that you disapprove of her actions; tell her that while she may have feelings of anger toward her brother, you are displeased with her expressions of pleasure at his misfortune. While it may take a long time to reverse the trend that now exists, you must do what you can to reassure her that she holds a very special place in your heart and that such hostility toward her brother is unnecessary and unwarranted.

I would like to underline that I believe problems of this sort can be prevented if parents plan their families so that the children are at least three years apart in age — and if they avoid making comparisons between the children at any stage in their development.

🍃

Sibling Relationships

My nine-year-old daughter has always worshipped her older brother. He seemed to enjoy her admiration; they got along well and loved doing things together. But now he is thirteen, and things have changed. At times he makes fun of his sister and tells her to "get lost" when she follows him around, particularly when he is with his friends. Does his age have something to do with this behavior? How can I explain the change to my daughter? How should I handle the situation with my son?

Most likely, your son loves his little sister as much as ever. But their interaction will change now that he has reached that stage in life when he wants to prove his independence and maturity, especially to his peers. Friends' opinions are often as important as family opinions to an adolescent, and your son may feel he's not "cool" among his fellow teenagers if his younger sister follows him everywhere. Because they're not sure of their own individuality, people your son's age form cliques, and in such groups they may show a tendency to bully or belittle others. You can imagine what his friends say when his nine-year-old sister accompanies him places; they probably tease him and make fun of her.

Of course this change will be confusing and painful for your daughter, and she will need your help in understanding that her brother is growing up and building a wider social circle for himself that still includes the family but now extends beyond it. Point out to her that "teenagers need time alone and time with other teenagers" and that she can't tag along with her brother as before. Acknowledge her feelings of hurt and disappointment, but explain that when she becomes a teenager, she'll realize that having a younger brother or sister always in tow might prove embarrassing and limit her activities.

You shouldn't belittle your daughter's feelings, nor should you be harsh with your son. At some point when you and he are communicating warmly and frankly, tell him that although *you* are pleased with his desire to show his independence, his adoring little sister is having some trouble with it. Certainly he should understand how keen are her hurt and embarrassment when he tells her to "get lost," and he must deal with her more delicately. If your son is responsive to your comments, you might ask him to spend a few minutes with his little sister when he is at home, since they now go out together less frequently. He may enjoy doing it more than he admits. Siblings often drift apart when one of them goes through a significant change, only to rediscover each other with new appreciation at later stages in their development.

❦

Teenage Family Responsibility

My mother keeps asking me to take care of my little brother and sister (they're five and seven years old). I'm twelve, and I have to watch them a lot on Friday and Saturday nights, sometimes until late. My mother says it's my responsibility, but I think it isn't fair. What should I say to her?

I agree with you — it isn't fair for you to have to take on so much of your parents' responsibilities. However, I do believe it's important for everyone in a family to cooperate in handling family responsibilities and to share in the work as well as the pleasures of family life. I'm sure you agree that from time to time you should help out by watching your brother and sister, but it is unfair for your parents to assume that you'll always be there to do it on a weekly basis. I suggest that you discuss this with your mother and let her know that you want to help out and share family responsibilities, but that doing this on a regular basis every weekend is causing you to resent it. Suggest to her you'd like to have some choice in the matter, that you would like her to discuss it with you in advance and get your approval.

I think it's as important for parents to respect the rights and feelings of children as it is for children to show similar respect toward their parents. I'm sure that if you were consulted about the matter in this way, you'd be cooperative, and actually appreciate helping your family out.

❧

Sibling Privacy

Our sons are eight and eleven now, and because of our financial situation and the size of our house, it's necessary for them to share a room. Is this damaging to each child's sense of individuality and privacy? Just how important is it for children to have separate rooms? If they must share a room, are there guidelines I should lay down for the sharing of the room?

There is absolutely nothing wrong with children sharing a room. It's not only a necessity in many families but it can work in a positive way to sensitize children to the individuality and rights of others.

117

The success of this situation, of course, depends upon how you handle it. To begin with, it's essential for you to respect the individuality of each child, and this can best be done by bringing your children into the decision-making process right from the beginning. Explain that the family's financial situation is something in which they have to share. Tell them that you would obviously like to give each his own room but that it simply isn't possible at this time — and make it clear that you want to work this all out in a way that makes it harmonious for everyone. Don't hesitate to ask their advice on how they would solve the problem if they were in your position. Children are basically compassionate and can understand problems better if you suggest that they imagine they are the person with the problem. Listen to the suggestions your children come up with, and do your best to implement them. If the room is large enough, you might consider installing a sliding wall or a screen so that it can be divided if they so desire from time to time. It's always helpful if each child can have a cabinet, closet, or dresser that can be locked; this reaffirms everyone's acknowledgment of the need for privacy in general and gives each one a "hideaway" in particular. You also might consider ways in which the boys can use other parts of the home for some of their special activities, such as homework, visiting with friends, or maintaining a hobby. This could cut down the chances for friction developing within the confines of their room. But prepare yourself for the fact that in such crowded circumstances, problems *are* bound to develop, and you will have to mediate from time to time.

In spite of the problems that are bound to erupt, I truly believe that children who are forced to share because of family circumstances frequently come away much more sensitive to the needs of others. They develop skills that will serve them in later years when they have to establish a harmonious life with another human being.

❦

The Biting Toddler

My two-year-old daughter seems to love children who are older or younger; however, when playing with children close to her own age, she tends to do a lot of biting and pinching. Is this something she will simply "grow out of"? What is the best way to handle this problem? Should I give her a pinch to show her how it feels?

Pinching and biting are things I totally disapprove of, even in the case of a two-year-old who is going through a stage in which it is normal to be crude in the expression of feelings, particularly toward children her own age. If you ignore her behavior, she will think it has your approval. And if you pinch or bite her back to "show her how it feels," you will be condoning this kind of behavior!

The best approach is to clearly show your disapproval by your facial expression and the tone of your voice. Then remove your daughter from the situation immediately, and tell her firmly that she cannot play with other children if she is going to bite and pinch. After a reasonably short time, allow her to go back to her playmates. If she misbehaves in this way a second time, remove her from the situation again. However, this second time keep her away from the other children even longer, to further emphasize the seriousness of her actions.

In all likelihood, this problem will subside quickly if you act in this way. But under no circumstances should you wait for your daughter to "grow out of it." Once this sort of behavior begins and is ignored, for even a short period of time, it is extremely difficult to stop.

❦

Unhappy Being Alone

I have a six-year-old son who is well liked by his peers, considered by his teachers to be a leader, and is generally a child who thrives when he's in a group. His problem seems to be his inability to amuse himself in solitary play. I've tried forcing him to stay in his game-filled room until he can find something to do, but he keeps coming out to pester me, and I end up playing games or doing projects with him. Does this behavior indicate that there is something wrong?

It sounds to me as if your six-year-old is a normal, outgoing child who simply enjoys being with other people more than he enjoys being by himself. When you really get down to it, being able to get along with other people is one of the most essential aspects of a healthy, happy life; and it sounds to me as if your son is well on the way to being a friendly, well-adjusted person. I don't think you should push such a natural extrovert into solitary play. It will only cause him to be unhappy and avoid solitude even more. In all likelihood, as he gets older his interests and inclinations will shift periodically, and he may go through phases when he actually enjoys being by himself.

I am glad to hear that you have participated in so many games and projects with him, and I hope you continue to do so. If you feel, however, that you need some relief, you might try to find a play group or some other community program that will provide him with both the peer relationships and the adult leadership that will satisfy his needs.

❧

Bossy Child

I'm worried about the way my four-year-old daughter interacts with other children her age. Whenever she is playing with them, she becomes very loud and bossy, and it seems as though she must always be the center of attention. She also can be very selfish at times, refusing to share her games and toys. Does this behavior mean my daughter will have trouble making — and keeping — friends later? Can she really be as antisocial as this behavior suggests, or is this normal for children her age?

If your daughter continues to behave this way, in all likelihood she *will* have trouble making and keeping friends later on in life. Sooner or later she will run into children who won't tolerate her self-centered behavior and who will turn to others for support and companionship. But it may take her some time to realize this, and so it is your job to let her know that other children will stop playing with her — and parents will keep their children away from her — if she continues to behave in this way. I don't suggest that you be overly critical of her behavior. Instead, let her know the consequences of her actions, and at the same time point out ways in which she can enjoy herself without taking such a dominant attitude. Don't hesitate to ask her to apply the golden rule — "How would you like it if other children treated you this way?"

My experience tells me that some children become bossy from time to time in an effort to try out different social approaches to other children. More often than not, they too become docile when they are faced with another overbearing child. By trying out different behavior patterns, children learn about themselves, as well as about the boundaries of acceptable social behavior. Unless a child is emotionally disturbed or harbors underlying feelings of inadequacy or weakness, he or she quickly abandons loud and overbearing attitudes on encountering other children who won't put up with that kind of "nonsense."

Helping Choose Your Child's Friends

After school and on weekends, my ten-year-old boy plays with other boys his age on our block, but I don't like them at all. They play very rough and wild and are nasty to adults and older children. I've told my son that I don't like him to associate with these boys, but he defends their behavior and says they're the only friends he has nearby. I'm afraid of the influence they'll have on my son, and I don't want them to lead him into trouble. Am I being overprotective? How strong can their influence actually be?

I don't think you're being overprotective, I think your concern is appropriate. Children — and for that matter, people of any age — are influenced by the company they keep. By all means encourage your son to spend time with those who respect others and have values of which you approve. However, he doesn't seem to have much of a choice other than isolating himself from all neighborhood friends.

Let him know that you are unhappy with the way in which his friends act toward other people and that you hope he will not copy their behavior. At the same time, let him know that you understand his need to play with other children, and acknowledge the fact that these boys are indeed his only companions close by. Look into the possibility of new friendships he might make — perhaps among his classmates or through some kind of boys' club, church group, or community organization. In the meantime, don't cut off his friendship with these other boys, but do do your best to communicate your feelings about their behavior. Caution your son about their influence, and work hard to find interesting alternatives to these neighborhood youngsters.

❦

Teenage Friendships

My fourteen-year-old daughter spends all her time with only one girl friend. The two of them don't participate in any group activities where they might meet other girls, and when they are not together, they're on the phone to each other. The girl is nice enough, but nothing special — and I feel they reinforce each other's tendencies toward shyness and withdrawal. Should I demand that she make other friends?

It is not uncommon for young people to pick a "best friend" and devote most of their time and attention to that person, and there are many advantages to a deep tie of this kind. In fact, some parents complain that their children don't relate strongly to one person and seem to respond only to group pressures.

Forming a deep friendship with one person is not as restricting or smothering as some people believe. Getting to know one person well and sharing many experiences with that person can sometimes be much more rewarding than just "hanging out" with a group. The fact that your daughter relates well to another human being in a meaningful relationship that is enjoyable and mutually gratifying is in itself mature and healthy behavior.

I don't think you should interfere — teenagers generally become rebellious when attempts are made to force them to carry out parental wishes — but at the same time I don't feel you should hesitate to let your daughter know what your feelings are. Suggest, but do not demand, that she see other boys and girls from time to time, simply so that she can get to know new people and broaden her experiences and interests. If you and your daughter both can communicate your feelings while respecting each other's individuality, this will open the possibilities for growth in her future, as well as in the future between the two of you.

Restricted Clubs

Our local high school has "clubs" that are much like sororities and fraternities. They go through a process of choosing certain "popular" students for membership while rejecting others. Both my teenagers, a son and a daughter, are talking about wanting to join. Can such groups be beneficial to young people? Or should I intervene and try to discourage them from getting involved?

Groups or clubs like this may enhance the self-esteem of those who are chosen to belong, but in my opinion it's a "self-esteem" that's based on the wrong criteria. When you really get down to it, what makes a membership so "elite" is its exclusiveness. Since a large number of people are rejected from membership, these clubs can make many people unhappy. They can also set apart the "elite" who are accepted into cliques that actually narrow the range of their experiences and give them a shallow and false sense of their own importance. In my mind, encouraging these kinds of clubs, fraternities, and sororities condones an exclusivity that runs counter to the spirit of human understanding — and an acceptance of people regardless of their individual differences — that is so necessary if we all are to live together in cooperation and peace.

As a parent, I don't think you should intervene, but I certainly think you should make a concerted attempt to convey to your teenagers the real meaning of such clubs and the potential harm they can do by causing emotional upset and feelings of rejection.

❦

Vandalism

My eleven-year-old was with a group of boys who were involved in some vandalism at school. They splashed paint over the school doorway and broke several windows. It turns out that our son was more on the sidelines of this than anything else. But he was present, and although he's contrite, he also doesn't seem terribly affected by what he and the others did. We don't want to make a federal issue out of this and make him feel riddled with guilt, but we also don't want to let this slide so that he thinks it's not that serious. And how do you answer a child when he says that "The others really did it, and I just went along"?

You must let your son know in no uncertain terms that this whole episode was a despicable act for which there is absolutely no excuse or justification. Make it clear that such vandalism is a serious disregard for other people's rights and property and that it could have escalated into an incident resulting in injury or even death. If a child *is* "riddled with guilt" over this sort of thing, it is much to everyone's advantage. It means the child has a conscience and can differentiate between what is right and what is wrong.

Let your son know that he, too was an active participant in this act of vandalism, regardless of how much damage he did or didn't do. The fact is that this was *his* group of friends and that he accompanied them on this pillage. Perhaps one of the most important ideas you have to get across to your son is that he should have taken an active part in trying to discourage the others; and if he realized he couldn't discourage them, he should have at least left the scene and not stood by to watch. His behavior, at best, indicates that he condoned what they did. Stress the importance of his role in trying to influence his peers when they are about to engage in destructive or unacceptable activities. He must understand that it is necessary for him to stand up for what he believes in, now and all the rest of his life. Finally, emphasize that people who keep bad company frequently end up in trouble themselves.

❦

The Child Who Doesn't Ask About Sex

My child is seven — and doesn't *ask about reproduction or sex. Should a parent talk to children about these things even if they don't broach the subject?*

Yes. Children have a natural curiosity about all things, and almost as soon as they can form sentences, most children begin to barrage their parents with questions on every conceivable subject. A child who doesn't ask questions about reproduction and sex by the time he or she is seven must have gotten the impression that this is a forbidden topic. Parents sometimes convey this attitude to children without being aware they are doing it — but children are extremely sensitive and pick up these things. On occasion, some adult may have passed their questions off by saying, "You're too young to know those things," or, "I never want to hear you ask questions like that." This sort of evasiveness may cause some children to suppress their natural questions about sex and reproduction, but their curiosity is still at work.

If children don't receive this sort of information from a concerned and reliable source, they may conjure up ideas that are not only far from reality and quite distorted but are also confusing and frightening, leaving them highly vulnerable to further mistaken notions about sexuality later on. For this reason, I believe you should be the one to broach the subject. Don't leave it to a stranger, a peer, or someone else whose interest in your child's welfare couldn't possibly match yours.

If you feel unqualified or unsure about how to discuss sexuality and reproduction with a young child, I suggest you consult books written by experts in the field of child psychology. Once you have broached the subject, your child will most likely respond with a number of questions to which you'll want to provide thoughtful, accurate answers.

❦

Teenage Sex Talk and Pornography

My fourteen-year-old is obviously very interested in sex — he and his friends look at magazines that contain erotic photographs, and I hear them discussing "dirty" movies and girls they'd like to "score" with. I don't know whether this interest in pornography is healthy, or what commentary a parent should make about this sort of thing. Should I just remain silent, or should I try to influence my son's ideas in some way?

If these discussions take place openly in your presence, you have a perfect right to enter into the conversations and express a judgmental attitude about their views.

The emergence of your son's sexual feelings understandably arouses his interest in erotic photographs and movies. Let your son know that both boys and girls have a natural and pleasurable interest in sex, but that "scoring" is a term that implies winning in competition. Sex is not a way to overwhelm others with their exploits, and if your son thinks of it in such a way, it will someday detract from the feelings of mutual gratification that are so rewarding in a sexual experience.

Your son's interest in sex is perfectly healthy and requires not only understanding on your part but a willingness to offer honest answers to any questions he may have — and to help him express his sexuality in a more respectful and responsible manner.

❧

Body Changes in Pre-Teenager

My eleven-year-old daughter's figure is beginning to develop, and although we have not actually discussed this, it seems to me she must feel very awkward about it. Should I make a point of discussing this with her — or leave it up to her to say something? How should a mother handle these sensitive new developments?

You are just assuming that she is sensitive about the changes in her body because she hasn't discussed them with you. You might be surprised to find that she is not the least bit sensitive about it; in fact, her silence might be in response to *your* awkwardness.

Unless you have somehow conveyed the idea that this is an unacceptable subject, your daughter would have asked all kinds of questions by now. Since she hasn't, I think you should be the one to speak up. Comment, in as casual a manner as you can, on the fact that she is growing up and that her body is and will be changing in a number of normal and natural ways. (If you haven't talked about menstruation yet, this is a good time to bring it up). Encourage her to talk to you about her feelings, and do not moralize or be judgmental about what she might tell you. Don't try to tell her that she shouldn't be so "sensitive" or "embarrassed"; instead, let her know that her feelings are nothing to be ashamed of, and that many teenagers and preteenagers feel self-conscious about the changes that take place in their bodies as they go from childhood to adulthood. By indicating your understanding and support, you can instill in her a sense of trust so that she can later turn to you with further questions.

❧

Preparation for Parenthood Programs for Teenagers

Members of our PTA have been talking about starting a program in the local high school that would help teenagers prepare for the problems of parenthood with which they'll probably have to deal someday. Our group of parents, though, is divided about the usefulness of such a program, and we'd appreciate hearing your reaction to the project. Do you think young people would really profit from exposure to such a subject? Is such a program necessary or helpful to them?

There is absolutely no doubt in my mind that young people of both sexes would benefit enormously from such educational programs. In fact, I consider this to be one of the most important projects a school — or for that matter, any local group — can undertake to help prevent emotional problems for future generations. I personally have devoted a great deal of energy to this subject because I believe that parents, and young people who someday will become parents, are in the "front line" of the quest for mental health. If young people have adequate and realistic information about the responsibilities of parenthood, they can make thoughtful choices about whether they wish to become parents, and they will have the background and knowledge necessary for them to become responsible parents.

129

This need for parent education is so profound that The National Foundation – March of Dimes has undertaken a national effort to support parent education by making information available to PTAs and various other community groups throughout the United States. For this purpose, and at their request, I myself have prepared three audio cassette tapes entitled "Conversations on Being a Parent." You can get these tapes, which cover six separate topics, by sending fifteen dollars to the Supply Division of The National Foundation – March of Dimes, Box 2000, White Plains, New York 10602.

❦

Discussing Sex with Children

I know I should take my children aside and talk to them about sex, but I feel terribly unsure about the manner or the language to use. What sort of words or examples are best? And after you've explained about something, how do you keep the lines of communication open for further discussion? Also, when do you talk to children? Is there a "right" time for talking about sex?

If you're open and frank with your children in answering questions about reproduction and sex without giving them the feeling that there's something "wrong" about discussing the subject, you've done all you can to show that the "lines of communication" are open. Assure your child that you'll always be available to explain things if questions arise. If parents are "matter-of-fact" with each other in discussing sexual matters, children pick up the tone of their parents' communication and will then be "matter-of-fact" themselves about future questions. If you're inhibited about the subject, you can be sure your children will sense it and be reluctant to discuss their concerns with you. At the same time, don't go overboard and bring up sexual matters each time you sit down to dinner simply to show your children that you are "with it." And *don't* badger them into discussing sexual matters if they don't want to. It's best to use words that are clear, understandable, and free of vulgar or demeaning connotations. Words that are biologically descriptive — words such as penis, vagina, ovary, and uterus — are far better than words that are "cute" or evasive (such as "down there" or "special place"). If you are straightforward and matter-of-fact in a relaxed way, and avoid any implications of lewdness or vulgarity, your child will find it easier to understand the details of sex and be less inclined to come away confused and reluctant to ask further questions, or be overly stimulated by provocative remarks. Don't hesitate to mention to your child, however, that some people do use other words that you consider "dirty" to describe parts of the body and sexual functions. If you say to your children that "I am sure you've heard some of these words, haven't you?" they may respond with some of the language they *have* heard. You can then clarify the meaning of these words and at the same time let your children know how you feel about them.

There's really no *right* time to talk to children about sex except when they raise questions. Perhaps when some issue arises on a television program, or when some news item appears that arouses everyone's interest, it can serve as a springboard for discussion. News of the birth of the first "test-tube baby," for instance, provoked many questions from children. Discussions about sex should take place in the same context as other discussions. During my professional practice as a psychologist, I've been appalled at the number of adult patients who have reported that "when the time came," their parents "took them aside" into the bathroom to tell them about sexual matters. By conducting this discussion in a separate room — particularly the bathroom — these parents conveyed to their children the idea that they considered sex forbidden and vulgar. When sexual matters are dealt with in this way, it not only can lead to sexual dysfunction later on in life but can lay the groundwork for distorted ideas about sex. And it can lead to more preoccupation with the issue that would otherwise be natural.

❦

Parental Sex and Their Children

My son and daughter-in-law make a point of being free and open sexually in front of their children, ages six and eight. They talk with them freely about intercourse, telling them that "Mommy and Daddy do it," and they are very casual about being nude in front of the children. I fear that children will be overstimulated by such an emphasis on sex at such a young age. Isn't this "too much too soon," and won't it distort their values? Or "scare" them by giving them more information than they're able to handle? How frank should parents be with their children about their own sexuality?

This all depends on how free these parents are and how they discuss these issues. As I read your question, I cannot help but wonder what your own values are. Some people who are extremely inhibited themselves find any casual reference to sexual matters as being "too free" or "too provocative." As a general rule, it's better for children to be "over" informed than it is for them to be underinformed.

I don't believe that parents should describe the details of their own sexual intercourse to their children, but I see nothing wrong with parents responding affirmatively to a child's question about whether "you and Daddy do it." Children who know that their own parents have a loving sexual relationship will have positive role models for their own future. I've known some youngsters, however, who have said, "Next time you do it, I

want to watch." This is the time to explain that sexual intercourse is a private matter, one that happens between two
people who want to be together.

I've always advocated that parents be casual with their children about nudity. On the other hand, I don't recommend that
parents be exhibitionists, walking about in a provocative manner. Children in the course of their own growth will develop
feelings of modesty not only about themselves but about their
parents. So, even though you may have started out being casual
with toddlers and preschoolers, you may eventually find that
your children prefer to leave the room when you're nude, or
close the door when they're undressing or bathing. This does
not mean that your child has become inappropriately inhibited
as a result of an underlying emotional problem. It merely is a
stage that all children go through.

For the most part, children themselves express shyness and
embarrassment when parents talk "too much" about sexual
matters, and these feelings should be respected. If more "openness" than children can handle is forced upon them, they may
react by becoming *more* inhibited rather than less.

❧

Coarseness About Sex

*My husband and I are concerned about the rather frank and
even insensitive and coarse attitude toward sex that seems
prevalent in young people today. I even overheard my daughter
and her friends refer to intercourse using some four-letter
words as part of their vocabulary. What do you say to teenagers today to make them realize the responsibilities of sex?
How do you impart values and mature attitudes to your children?*

The concern you and your husband have about the insensitivity and coarseness that your children seem to have about sex is understandable. However, your children may be expressing their peers' attitudes more than their own. It's not at all uncommon for young people, particularly when they're anxious about something, to compensate for their anxiety with an air of superiority or bravado. The use of four-letter words to refer to intercourse is not only common but it's somewhat understandable when you stop to consider how "word poor" our language is when it comes to sexual matters. There is a gap in our language because of our social taboos in this area, a gap that has unfortunately been filled by colloquial expressions and vulgarities.

As a parent, you should not hesitate to let your children know of your displeasure about their insensitivities, coarseness, or vulgar expressions. However, I don't think you should try to suppress children completely. Let them know you much prefer to hear them discuss their feelings in less vulgar or provocative terms.

It's hard to teach teenagers about their responsibilities of sex and to impart attitudes of respect about sexual feelings unless you've had a trusting relationship with them right from the start. If you've answered their questions honestly and been a responsive parent whenever their needs arose, they will respect you and your ideas, your values and feelings. But if sex has been taboo, or if you've been punitive when children have used certain expressions or raised questions about sexuality, in all likelihood they will have turned elsewhere for guidance in the development of their sexual attitudes.

❧

Parental Embarrassment in Discussing Sex

My adolescent daughter doesn't talk to me about sex, although I hear that she talks to others. This only serves to make me feel even more inadequate about my own embarrassment and confusion as a parent in matters concerning my child's sexual guidance. Have I failed my child in some way?

I wouldn't exactly call it a failure, but I would say that your embarrassment and confusion have obviously been conveyed to your daughter in a way that makes it difficult for her to discuss sexual matters with you. You are by no means alone. Many parents find themselves in the same situation.

Your daughter clearly finds it more comfortable to talk to other people — in all likelihood, her peers — about her emerging sexual interests. It is to be hoped that her friends are knowledgeable enough and will help her develop healthy attitudes about sexual matters. Your situation is a clear demonstration of what happens when parents, for one reason or another, are unable to discuss sexuality at an earlier age. Young people in situations like this are far more vulnerable to forces outside the family influencing their sexual attitudes than are youngsters whose parents are casual and open in their discussions of sexuality.

Parental Explanations of Wet Dreams and Menstruation

Our thirteen-year-old son is beginning to have nocturnal emissions — wet dreams. I feel that this should be discussed with him, and I asked my husband to do so. Although my husband agreed, he comes home from work exhausted and "doesn't get around to it" and says, "You tell him." He also says that since our son hasn't asked about the wet dreams himself, we should "wait until he mentions it." Is he right? Should parents let well enough alone about these things till children ask about them? (Our eleven-year-old daughter has never asked about menstruation either.) And should mothers be the ones to talk to their sons, or should I insist that my husband get more involved?

No, I don't think you should simply wait until your son mentions it. I think you should discuss with both your children the physical and emotional changes that you know take place as children approach their teenage years. If children have prior knowledge and understanding of these events, they will not be as disconcerting or even frightening as they might be if they are caught unawares.

It is generally assumed that fathers should talk to sons and mothers to daughters. I don't necessarily agree with this. I believe it's far better if parents can feel free to discuss sexual matters with their children regardless of their gender. Nevertheless, mothers *do* sometimes have difficulty discussing sexual matters with their sons and fathers with their daughters. In your case, it might be best for both your children to be involved with you and your husband together in a general discussion of the changes that take place around the teenage years for both boys and girls.

Find a time when everyone is in a pleasant mood and bring the matter up casually. Explain that as boys mature, semen — a white sticky substance that has sperm in it — is stored in their testicles. When they have sexual dreams that are exciting, it can cause them to ejaculate semen in their sleep. Let your son know that it's normal and part of growing up. In the same manner, let your children know that as a girl's body matures, the ovaries begin to produce tiny eggs that, once a month, go from the ovary to the Fallopian tube into the uterus; then, if the egg is not fertilized by a sperm, it leaves the body. Explain that this causes a flow of blood that takes place once each month for a few days. An excellent book I would recommend as a guide for parents to help their children understand these specific problems is entitled *Girls Are Girls and Boys Are Boys, So What's the Difference?* This book was written by Dr. Sol Gordon and is well illustrated. It's published by John Day Company of New York.

🍎

Teenagers and Birth Control

I hear so much about teenagers and sex that I worry about my own teenagers — a daughter, fourteen, and a son, sixteen. I wonder if I should say something to them about birth control and the responsibilities of intercourse, but by doing so, I don't want to put ideas in their heads that might not otherwise be there, or make it seem that I condone their becoming sexually active.. Should I talk to my children? And how should I do so without making it seem I sanction their sexual activity?

Merely knowing about sexual matters and birth control does not cause young people to go out and experience these things for themselves. The fact is that teenagers today have opportunities to become sexually involved regardless of whether or not you "put ideas in their heads." And parents have the right and responsibility to see that those "ideas" include their own feelings and values about sexual matters. My experience has shown that young people who receive information and guidance from parents whom they trust are far less likely to get into sexual difficulty than young people whose parents failed to become involved in the transmission of sexual information. By displaying a sense of knowledgeable concern and responsibility in educating their children, parents provide a model of what responsibility really is.

A discussion of these matters is not as difficult as you might think. Simply and frankly convey to your children the emotional implications and possible consequences of sexual activity. Explain to them that when two people have sexual relations, deep feelings of emotional intensity are often involved. Let them know how important it is, in situations where intercourse might possibly occur, to be sensitive to the other person's feelings and to respect his or her reactions and wishes — but at the same time to stand up for their own feelings of what is right or what their own wishes are. Explain that if pregnancy should occur — and this will be entirely possible if appropriate precautions are not taken — it will mean dealing with an even greater complexity of feelings and responsibilities, at a time in their lives when they should be free to grow and explore a variety of possibilities for their own future.

Let them know that you will always be available to talk to them about any matters that trouble them on this subject — and if specific situations arise in which they think it would be helpful to know more about birth-control procedures, you will discuss it with them. Make it clear that while you feel it's important to inform them about birth control and sexual responsibility, you are not suggesting that you think it's right for them to become sexually active at present, but that you think it will be helpful for them to begin to be aware of these matters at this time in their lives.

❦

Nightmares

About six months ago, we had a bad fire in our house. Although no one was injured, my four-year-old still wakes up at night screaming that something is on fire. We've explained to him that everything is all right and that there is no more fire, but these nightmares persist. Is this normal? What should we do?

His nightmares are certainly understandable in view of the alarming event that occurred. Generally speaking, children do have nightmares after frightening experiences, and as time goes on, the dreams tend to diminish in frequency. If your son has nightmares perhaps once or twice a month, I would say this is normal for his age. If, however, he continues to have recurrent nightmares about fire, and these occur several times a week, professional help may be advisable. With some children, a traumatic event may cause an underlying emotional problem to surface and may make a child's reaction to an upsetting event even more intense. As time goes on, it is no longer the traumatic event that the child is reacting to, but the emotional problems that were there all along and that were, in a sense, triggered and brought to the surface by the traumatic event.

❦

Fear of Water

My nine-year-old has what seems to me an abnormal fear of water. All the rest of our family enjoy swimming, but no matter how much we try to coax her into the water or insist that she take swimming lessons, she refuses to even try. (When her brother, who's a year older, teases her and tries to pull her into the water, she screams and runs away.) Are some children simply born with a fear of water? What can we do to help her overcome her fears?

Children are not born with a fear of water. In fact, evidence shows that newborn infants have reflex reactions that would enable them to swim if necessary. In a sense, they have developed in an aquatic environment in their first nine months of life prior to birth. Also, it is thought by many that a growing fetus goes through all the phases of evolution that led up to the specialized behavior characteristic of humans, and that includes a phase where an unborn child has the qualities of an aquatic species.

All of this is a somewhat academic explanation of a newborn's natural propensity for water. Obviously, your daughter has had some experience in her life that has caused her to develop her fears. The truth is that a bath for a young child can be as frightening as it can be pleasurable. Many young children have been accidentally doused in a tub or have been inadvertently terrorized during a hair washing by soap that stings their eyes. It may take just a few such frightening experiences, close together in time, to convince a child that water is frightening and something to be avoided at all costs.

Once children become frightened in this way, it takes a great deal of patience and tolerance to help them overcome it. When such a reaction appears during infancy or early childhood, it is important to try to overcome the fears as quickly as possible and do what you can to make bath time "fun."

Obviously, coaxing or pressuring your daughter does not work. Teasing her or trying to pull her into the water is even worse. I think you should encourage her to take swimming lessons with a patient and understanding teacher. Do not insist upon it — any pressure on her will cause her to recoil even more — but offer this to her as an opportunity to learn something she will enjoy, and indicate your understanding of her anxieties and fears.

Children frequently learn better from each other than they do from grownups or experts. Try to find a friend your daughter admires who can quietly help her. Children of your daughter's age often admire teenagers, so a friend or acquaintance who is thirteen or fourteen might have sufficient influence to help her overcome her fears.

❧

Helping with Monsters Under the Bed

My four-year-old is absolutely terrified of the "witches and monsters" she says are under her bed — and just about the time I think she's gone to sleep for the night, she'll start crying that she's "afraid of the witch" or she "hears the lion," and I'll have to go in to comfort her. My husband says that we shouldn't go in to her when she acts like this, that our comforting her only encourages her fantasies. He thinks we should just tell her that "these things aren't real, she's acting silly," and that's that. He also thinks she's at an age where she no longer needs a night light in her room. Why do children believe in these imaginary monsters? And how should we handle the situation?

No matter how imaginary the witches, lions, and monsters are to you and your husband, they are *very* real to your daughter. You might succeed in convincing her that witches and monsters are not actually under her bed at the moment, but in her mind they are ever-present and can move from place to place at the flick of an eye. All the reasoning in the world won't make these imaginary, scary things go away because their existence is in the child's mind and not in the real world. When your child is frightened and crying out, she needs comfort and compassion. Ignoring her will only intensify her fears.

Children don't simply believe in imaginary monsters for the adventure of it; they would willingly annihilate them or banish them from their fantasies if possible. No matter how imaginary the monsters are, the feelings within the child from which they are derived are not at all imaginary. Those witches and monsters are expressions of those angry, hostile, and aggressive feelings that actually originate within the child. Early in life, children have trouble channeling their hostile and aggressive feelings, or expressing them in a socially acceptable way. They are left with the choice of letting these feelings come out without restraint, which they cannot do without risk of hurting those they love, or transforming these feelings into bad and evil things, which express those unacceptable emotions for them. In effect, the child is saying that it's not *me* who's doing bad and horrible things — it's the witch or the monster who does bad, nasty things to *me*.

In general, these fears in children are transitory and eventually go away as a child learns to come to terms with his or her hostility or anger. In the meantime, offer comfort and support and help your child deal with feelings about the monsters rather than try to convince her that the monsters don't exist.

As far as a night light is concerned, if it helps a child sleep more comfortably and feel less frightened, I see no reason not to use one. Even many adults like a little light somewhere in the room when they go to sleep, if for no other reason than to help them get oriented if they wake suddenly at night.

❦

The Untalkative Child

My three-year-old seems bright, alert, and physically healthy — but he rarely speaks! He expresses his needs and wants in short phrases, but doesn't ask questions and talk freely like other three-year-olds. His six-year-old brother is a real chatterbox. Could this be the reason for our son's quiet ways? How can we get him to speak more often?

I have seen children who simply can't get a word in edgewise because their parents talk a great deal. But it's not likely that a sibling would cause this to happen. It sounds to me as if you simply have two different children with two different personalities. Children not only vary in personality and temperament right from the start, but they also have different developmental patterns. Some children start out speaking very little, but ultimately become very talkative as they grow from one stage into another. Others may be very noisy right from the start and continue on that way.

My thirteen-year-old daughter, Pia, was basically a quiet child and one who didn't talk freely to strangers. While she was not withdrawn — she was in fact quite friendly — she just didn't say very much. I wasn't the least bit concerned, but other people commented on her shyness. I was convinced this would change as she grew — and indeed it did! To say that today she is highly verbal is an understatement! In fact, I once in exasperation said, "Pia, please, can't you be quiet for a while and let other people speak?" She said, "I can't help it, every time I try, the words keep coming out anyway."

In all likelihood, your son will in time emerge with a verbal facility that may make you wonder why you ever complained about his quietness!

❦

Teenager Who Hoards His Money

While other kids are squandering money on comic books and candy, our thirteen-year-old hoards his allowance, keeping track of every penny and even charging other children interest on money they borrow from him! At first we thought his tight-wad tactics were amusing, but lately we feel his penny-pinching has gone too far. Should we be alarmed? What could cause him to behave this way?

Frankly, I think your son's behavior is extreme. If his primary pleasure seems to come from hoarding his allowance, he is indeed being overly miserly.

While I don't think you should be alarmed about this, it is important for you to try to influence his current ideas about money. Encourage your son to be more flexible. Let him know that you think some of his money should be used for his own enjoyment — and that some of these pleasures can be shared with friends. Let him know that charging interest on money he lends is hardly a friendly gesture, and can even cause him to be rejected by others.

Strange as it may seem, your son's miserly attitude about money could have its origins in the way he was toilet trained. When toilet training is conducted in a coercive manner, and when parents seem to place excessive importance on the process, children sometimes develop feelings of resistance about parting with something that adults obviously regard with great significance. Under such circumstances, a child sees that "holding back" gives him a sense of power in dealing with adults. As he matures, he may unconsciously transfer this withholding tendency to another "product" that adults seem to value — in this case, money.

❦

The Extremely Modest Child

My nine-year-old is so modest that it's almost an obsession with her. If anyone is around when she's dressing or undressing, she goes to ridiculous lengths to keep herself covered, squealing if I come near. Do all youngsters of this age go through phases of such pronounced modesty?

This is not at all uncommon, though generally speaking, it occurs at an earlier age than your daughter's. Whatever you do, don't embarrass her or make fun of her. Don't insist that she undress in front of you or belittle her in any way. You might try being more casual about your own nudity to reinforce the idea that being seen dressing or undressing is nothing to be ashamed or embarrassed about.

In the course of establishing their own identity, children frequently depart from their parents' attitudes and views in an attempt to try things their own way. This does not mean they are rejecting you or rebelling against you. They are simply asserting themselves in their attempt to discover how they want to handle their own lives. Your daughter will eventually work things out her own way, and her extreme modesty is likely to be replaced by an attitude or behavior pattern more closely akin to your own.

❦

Curiosity About Handicapped People

While my five-year-old daughter and I were waiting for a bus, she very loudly asked me why the lady next to us, who had come down the street from the school for the blind, was using a long white cane. "She looks funny," my child said loudly. My daughter has done this before from time to time when she has seen someone who looks strange to her, asking me in public why a handicapped person "acts queer" or "looks different." Are children just blatantly insensitive? What should I say to her?

This is *not* insensitivity on the part of children, it is simply the result of their natural naiveté and truthfulness. Children quickly pick up details that make one person or situation different from another, and they question those differences in order to learn more about the world and people in it. You need to explain in concrete detail what these unfamiliar things mean. Simply explain to your daughter that blind people use a cane to help guide them as they walk so that they will not bump into other people or objects or walk off curbs into traffic. Do not hesitate to offer this explanation on the spot, in conversational tones, in front of the person involved. (If you express obvious embarrassment at your child's remarks and attempt to answer her questions in a shocked whisper, it can only serve to make a handicapped person feel stigmatized and upset, and to make your child feel there is something frightening and wrong about what is happening.) Then, sometime later, when you are alone with your daughter, point out that while her remarks at that moment were not meant to hurt anyone, it is often better to wait until another time and place for such questions, to avoid the possibility of hurting someone's feelings.

In my experience, people with handicaps appreciate being dealt with in as casual and open a way as possible. A compassionate and unflustered attitude on your part will help your child learn respect for each person's feelings and individuality, and also will serve as a model for your daughter in dealing with handicapped people now and later in her life.

❦

Helping Understand About Handicapped Sibling

Our three-year-old was born prematurely, and it's becoming sadly and increasingly clear as he gets older that he suffered some brain damage that will make him slow in both his physical and mental development, and that he will require special attention and education on our part. How do we explain their brother's handicaps to our other chidren, who are six and nine? What do we say to the other children in the neighborhood?

All children should be brought up to respect the individuality of others, whether it involves differences that are racial, religious, physical, or psychological. I think you should be open and direct with your other children — and with their playmates in the neighborhood — in discussing the abilities and limitations of your three-year-old. Explain his special situation as best you can, and ask for their help in dealing with it. Tell them you will always be available to answer questions about any problems that arise, and explain that even though their brother gets a great deal of attention, you are as deeply interested in what is happening to the two of them. Your attitude will not only demonstrate your acceptance of each individual family member but will help everyone deal with the problems and pressures that may arise.

By avoiding the subject or by being secretive about your child's limitations, you help no one. In fact, you leave your son vulnerable to criticism and misunderstanding, and create an atmosphere of "shame" about any problems he has. Life is far more pleasant and rich when we can enjoy and learn from the differences among us. People with handicaps have a vision and a grace that is all their own. By teaching compassion to our children, we can help them be thankful for what they have and at the same time help them feel satisfaction and pride in offering their own resources and abilities to help others.

Helping Children
Understand Homosexuality

My nine-year-old daughter has been taking piano lessons for about a year now from a young man we all like very much. He loves music and has taught our daughter with real sensitivity and skill (I know because he comes to our house for the lessons, and I can hear what's going on). Yesterday she came home in tears because some older children had told her he was "gay" and lived with another man. She wants to know what this means, and why it is wrong. Should a parent explain homosexuality to a young child — and if so, how? Is there any reason to discontinue her lessons because of this?

It seems to me that this young man is not only an excellent teacher but a likable person with integrity and sensitivity who has gained your child's affection. I see no reason whatsoever for you to discontinue her piano lessons with him. I believe that as long as he doesn't broach the subject of his sexual preferences — whether heterosexual or homosexual — with your daughter, his personal life is his own business.

By all means answer your daughter's questions about homosexuality. Affirm the fact that human beings have a strong need to love and be loved, and to form attachments where this love can grow. Explain that homosexuals find greater satisfaction in having deep relationships with members of their own sex. Point out that some people who find this upsetting make fun of homosexuals but that all people should be allowed to make their own choices and should not be criticized or persecuted for the way they feel. During this discussion, explain words such as "gay," "homosexual," and "lesbian" so that she will be properly and sensitively informed about them. I feel that we should let children know that it is unfortunate when an individual is cruelly ridiculed, sometimes even discriminated against, because of personal preferences that do not harm anyone else. This is another way in which we can help our children develop compassion and sensitivity for people who are different.

❦

Readiness to Travel to School Alone

We live in a large metropolitan area, and our eight-year-old son goes to a city school. I think our child should ride the city buses by himself so that he will be encouraged to be more independent; my husband thinks he should be escorted to school by one of us. What do you think? When is a child old enough to ride on public transportation all alone?

I agree that your child should be encouraged to be independent; at the same time, he needs a certain degree of protection as he works toward this goal. If he is subjected to a situation where the probability of having a frightening experience is high, it could not only undermine his growing independence but could cause him to develop an inordinate fear of being out in the world alone.

In deciding when a child is old enough to use public transportation, you must take into consideration not only the child's age but also his or her personal degree of maturity, resourcefulness, physical size, and interest in undertaking this particular task. Independence comes from developing and using one's personal resources to deal with the demands of everyday life in a wide variety of situations — and traveling alone is only one of them. If there is a real risk that your child will be frightened, lost, or even threatened, it might be best to put off his traveling alone until he is physically bigger and has a greater sense of self-assurance about handling things on his own. Then, when your child is ready to take on this responsibility, he will let you know, and if you see that the dangers are minimal, by all means let him go.

❦

Threats to Run Away from Home

Often, after we have an argument, my six-year-old, furious that he can't have his own way, will announce that he's "running away from home." Why does a child do this? One mother I know always laughs at her son and says she'll help him pack. Is this a good approach? How should a parent handle this?

I don't think you should completely ignore the threat, and I certainly don't think you should "help your child pack." No child who threatens to run away really wants to go through with it. However, if you ignore or make fun of the threat, or if you go so far as to actually assist him in carrying it out, he may feel compelled to leave for no other reason than simply to save face.

Behind your child's thoughts of running away is a reassuring fantasy that he will be sorely missed by his family. In all likelihood, the fantasy includes a frantic search for him, feelings of great regret that he was ever criticized, a warm welcome upon his return, and the complete and unconditional acceptance of his terms for future behavior. I think that all children, whether they actually voice their threats to run away from home or not, have entertained similar fantasies when all was not going well in their lives at that moment. A child's common reaction is to feel that "nobody loves me, but just wait — when I'm gone, they'll be sorry." (This, incidentally, is not unlike the feelings and fantasies of a child who threatens suicide. Some troubled young people, unfortunately, believe that in some way they will be around to see their parents' remorse and grief, not really grasping the fact that they will not be present and will not be able to receive that satisfaction.)

When your son threatens to run away, it's best to react by explaining that you know he's angry with you and is unhappy about your anger toward him. Make it clear that being angry at him doesn't mean you don't love him. Assure him emphatically that your love is as strong as ever, even though you've just had an argument. Let him know that if he were to leave home, it would upset you terribly. Ask him to imagine how upsetting it would be if *you* left him and ran away simply because you had an argument. Don't present this as a threat, but as a statement of fact.

In my professional experience, I've found that most children who actually run away do so because their parents show little or no interest in discussing the feelings of discontent a child has about his life and family problems. The threat to run away should tell you that the child is in some way asking you to listen to him; he needs your assurance that, in spite of the differences or conflicts between you, he still has your deep love.

❦

Learning to Deal with the Outside World

Now that my daughter is twelve, I'd like her to help me by occasionally going to the store for groceries. She resists, saying that she's "scared someone will bother her" or that the grocer "won't know what she wants." I sometimes wonder if this is just an excuse for laziness. I don't want to force my child to do anything that frightens her, but I do think she should be learning to deal with the outside world. How should a parent handle this?

Your daughter's reaction is not uncommon, and in all likelihood, her fears will diminish as she gets older. In the meantime, try to give her the reassurance that she needs to venture away from home on her own. Don't push her out without any attempts at support or understanding, but on the other hand, don't be overly protective and allow her to avoid all responsibilities. If you do, she may learn that expressing such fears is a way to avoid dealing with new situations.

It is true for any of us, however, that new responsibilities may seem overwhelming when tackled all at once instead of in manageable stages bit by bit. Explain to your daughter that even adults learn to cope with new things a little at a time, and ask her to come along with you when you go to the store and shop for groceries. And have her become more familiar with other places you might send her on errands. As time goes by and she becomes more self-assured, she will be more willing to handle these tasks without you.

It's not totally unrealistic for a twelve-year-old to be afraid that she might be bothered by strangers. If you push her into the "outside world" while she has these fears, they will only become more intense, and her resistance will increase. Assure her that you understand that she's scared at times but that you know she will get over it. Your patient and understanding attitude will make it much easier for her to accept and develop her independence, which will then allow her to venture farther away from home and into situations of uncertainty.

As children grow, they vary in their degree of readiness for moving out alone into the world — but they'll generally let you know when they feel ready to take on new tasks. Until then, agree that some precaution with strangers is wise, but that as she gets older, she'll begin to get enjoyment and satisfaction out of meeting people and accomplishing tasks on her own. Your patient understanding and training will make it easier for her to handle the responsibility when the time comes.

❧

The Child with a Difficult Teacher

My child had a fine time in first grade. Now the second grade has started, and his grades aren't nearly as good. Although he doesn't complain, I can tell he doesn't particularly like his new teacher — and after the last PTA meeting, I can see why. She's not nearly as warm or encouraging as his teacher last year. How should a parent handle this?

I think you should be as open and direct with your child as possible. Explain to him that not all teachers are the same, that some are more friendly or more interesting — and interested in *him* — than others. Point out to him that throughout his life, no matter what sort of work he does, he will encounter some people he likes and others he likes less.

Whatever you do, acknowledge and accept his feelings about what he is going through, but do not be critical of his current teacher, other than to acknowledge the fact that she is different from the teacher he had before. If you are critical of her, you will undermine her position and contribute to a lack of motivation on your child's part. Let your son know that it may be more difficult for him to do as well as he did last year but that you know he is able to make a greater effort. If you focus your interest and attention on his efforts rather than his grades, you will be supporting his actual work without using his grades as criteria of success.

While I don't like to see children penalized because of the

personality characteristics of adults, particularly their teachers, it is nevertheless important for them to learn how to contend with situations that are difficult. No one's life is without some disappointment, and helping your child to learn to cope at this stage will help him deal with disappointments in the years ahead.

❦

Beauty Contests for Children

In our local grade school they hold beauty contests, sponsored by the PTA! We refused to allow our six-year-old daughter to compete this past year, even though she cried and pleaded, but now we face the prospect of her competing in other contests from baton twirling to foot races. We don't want to deny any of our children participation in school and recreational activities – but somehow, all of this seems wrong at her age. What do you think?

I agree that these competitive activities are completely unnecessary for a young child — and can even be harmful. A far greater problem for children is their inability to cooperate — a problem not just for children but for adults and nations as well. That is why I would prefer that schools emphasize cooperative activities that teach children to work together instead of encouraging them to compete with one another. Children should be praised and rewarded for their outstanding abilities and skills, but they should not be pitted against each other in such a way that one child's success will depend upon another child's failure. Such contests create tremendous pressure and anxiety for all the children involved and lead to a feeling of failure or a diminished self-esteem on the part of those who lose.

I feel that any competitive activities in a school situation should be conducted in a lighthearted manner, to avoid animosity. All children involved should be praised for their efforts. And exuberant adults should be careful not to let their own values take over, intensifying the competitive atmosphere to such a pitch that children are caught up in a bewildering contest of adult egos and standards of "success."

But while many competitive activities conducted in the right spirit and atmosphere can be enjoyable and rewarding for young people, I am unalterably opposed to "beauty" contests. First of all, no skill is involved — "success" depends upon the physical qualities a child is born with, qualities that are then judged on the basis of very arbitrary and personal tastes. I don't believe physical beauty should be emphasized as an important quality, and I believe you should make your feelings about this known to your PTA. You will face opposition, but as you talk to other parents, I'm sure you will find that others share your reactions and that you can work to change some of these activities.

In the meantime, let your daughter know how you feel about these competitive activities. Make it clear to her that you love her whether she wins or loses, and couldn't care less about her friends' "awards." I don't think you should literally prevent her from competing since it singles her out from her peers. You can, however, give her the support and guidance she needs in dealing with her feelings during these endeavors.

❦

Homework

Last Sunday night my ten-year-old did it again — she announced that she had "boring" homework to do, then pleaded with us to help her finish it. She consistently puts her school-

work off until the last minute, then calls on us for assistance, and it's become increasingly annoying. Why is she so undisciplined about this? Is there a way for us to deal with this procrastination? What can we say to her?

If your daughter tends to procrastinate about homework in particular, but assumes her responsibilities in most other areas of her life, in all likelihood her homework itself is the problem and not a lack of discipline in general. If homework is boring or uninteresting, even the most highly motivated child will find it unpleasant and will want to put it off for as long as possible. If this is the case, let her know that you understand her feelings about it, that you're aware it's not a pleasant task, but nevertheless it is one that simply has to be completed. Point out the advantages of getting an unappealing task over with so that it is no longer on her mind; explain that then she will be free to do other things without carrying around the burden of the unfinished homework. Announce the time at which you will be available to help her get started, then make an active effort to sit down, open the books, and begin work with her. But under no circumstances should you do the homework *for* her.

Nagging or threatening simply puts more pressure on her and makes things worse. Moreover, it places you in a position where you may be seen by your child as being dispassionate, uncooperative, and unconcerned about her dilemma. But by participating actively to help her with her problem, you are showing your understanding of her feelings, demonstrating a method for tackling an unpleasant task, and preventing that overwhelming panic a child feels when there is so little time and so much homework to do.

❦

Postpartum Depression

As time approaches for my baby to be born, I worry more and more about the postpartum depression that I've heard others talk about. My sister-in-law, for one, went into a real slump for weeks after her baby's birth. What is postpartum depression? Is there a real psychological or physical basis for it? Is there anything I can do to prepare myself for it?

Postpartum depression is an upsetting, overwhelming feeling that may strike a new mother suddenly, making her feel that she is helpless and unable to cope with her new baby. Some mothers feel so agitated and angry that they even have the impulse to run away from the families that now "entrap" them.

Postpartum depression does not affect all mothers in a severe way, but many new mothers experience it to some degree. Whether the feelings are mild or intense, postpartum depression can happen in the delivery room right after the birth of the baby or at any time during the first month following delivery. I find that it often happens on the fourth or fifth day following delivery or approximately one month after the baby is born — around the time the menstrual cycle is beginning to get back to normal.

For the most part, postpartum depression has a physical basis, even though the reaction is largely a psychological one. Hormone changes that have taken place in the mother gradually from the time of conception on to the delivery of the child have now undergone a sudden change. Estrogen and progesterone, which build up to a high level during pregnancy, drop very quickly right after delivery. This physical change can create a feeling of depression in itself. And if the woman has had an unusual amount of anxiety about becoming a mother, that psychological state together with the physical changes can combine to make a difficult time for a new mother.

In my own practice as a psychologist, I have also found that every mother I have known with a severe postpartum depression had given birth to a boy. It suggests even more strongly that hormone changes play the primary role in contributing to postpartum depression. During pregnancy, hormones from the baby pass through the placenta into the mother, and vice versa. If a mother is pregnant with a male child, her body will have become used to some male hormones, which will be stopped abruptly at the time of delivery. It seems very possible that this male hormone, called testosterone, may intensify the reaction even more.

The best way to cope with the depression is to take time to take good care of yourself. Get help with the care of your child and make an effort to get out and be with friends and indulge or enjoy yourself in whatever ways possible. Emotional support from your husband will be especially valuable at this difficult time, and will go a long way toward overcoming this unpleasant state.

It's important for every woman to know that postpartum depression is not at all uncommon and does not mean that a new mother is inadequate or ultimately unable to cope. It's a temporary physiological state caused by physical changes that have occurred as a result of your pregnancy and delivery. In most cases it subsides spontaneously, but if the discomfort is intense and leaves you incapable of assuming your responsibilities, don't hesitate to speak to your doctor and get the medical or psychological help you need.

❦

Childbirth, a Family Experience

My first child was born in a hospital where the medical care was first-rate — but where my family was relegated to the waiting room, and my baby was whisked off after delivery and it was several hours before I could cuddle it. Now I'm pregnant again and have heard of another hospital that is happy to cooperate with a couple who wants to have natural childbirth and that generally has facilities to make childbirth a more satisfying experience for the entire family. Is it worth switching to another hospital, even though it is a farther distance away, in order to give birth? What are your feelings about this matter?

Childbirth, in my opinion, should be viewed as a family experience and *not* merely a medical one. For more than twenty years I've been an advocate of family-centered childbirth — a process that focuses on the family as a unit and respects the feelings and dignity of the mother, the father, and the siblings. Every effort should be made to have the father participate in the labor and delivery of a child. Moreover, both parents should have sufficient knowledge about the possible procedures and medications involved in the delivery so that they will not only have knowledge about what may happen but will have some options in deciding what methods, techniques, and medication the mother chooses to have. A hospital that respects the integrity of the family unit and adapts itself to the emotional needs of all the family members serves to bring everyone within that family much closer and make the birth experience one of great joy and happiness.

Clearly, childbirth should be as satisfying an emotional experience as possible for the entire family. Hospital staffs should take into consideration the natural instincts human beings have and the protective feelings parents have toward their children. For instance, mothers have a real need to be close to their babies immediately following birth, and a mother's desire to nurse her newborn even in the moments just after birth in the delivery room should be given support by the medical staff. Even little brothers and sisters of the new baby should have the privilege and satisfaction of seeing their sibling and their mother as soon after birth as possible. In my experience, fathers who are actively involved in the labor and are present in the delivery room when their children are born are far more involved in caring for their children later on than fathers who have not been present at that critical time. I believe childbirth as a family experience serves to "imprint" on every family member the importance of the family as a functioning unit. The intense emotions surrounding the birth of a baby should be shared by everyone in the family — and should certainly be respected by members of the medical community.

In recent years there has been a trend for couples to want to have their babies born at home. I believe this trend has resulted from the general lack of humanism that exists in many hospitals' maternity units. Ideally, it's best for a baby to be born in an environment where any medical emergency can be dealt with promptly; at the same time, it's equally important for that environment to provide the optimal conditions supplying emotional support and respect for the feelings of the total family. It is certainly worth your time and effort to explore this matter with your doctor and with the hospitals in your community, to make sure your family's experience is as satisfying as possible. Even if this involves traveling a somewhat longer distance to reach the hospital of your choice, your ultimate experience should make the trip utterly worthwhile.

❦

False Pregnancy of Husband

Is there such a thing as a "sympathetic pregnancy"? I feel fine, but my husband wakes up nauseated, and says he's exhausted. It's as though he's picking up my symptoms. Is this possible — and why?

It's not only possible, it's even got a scientific name — it's called pseudocyesis. While it's not very common, some of the symptoms of pregnancy *are* occasionally reflected in an expectant father's behavior. Morning sickness, feelings of exhaustion, strange food cravings at weird hours of the night, and sometimes even abdominal swellings occur.

A number of years ago I had a male patient who did indeed have all these symptoms. In the course of his treatment, it became clear that he was jealous of the attention his pregnant wife was receiving, and his symptoms of "pregnancy" subsided only after he was able to face up to his fear of losing his wife's affection and his anger at the unborn child.

It's actually more common for women who are not pregnant to develop "sympathetic pregnancies," particularly when they have mixed feelings about having a child or have had difficulty in conceiving. Pseudocyesis is also a fairly common occurrence in animals. Cats and dogs will at times show physical signs of pregnancy and will "adopt" a small object or toy and nurse it as if it's an offspring. Animals may even lactate in order to "nurse" the supposed kitten or puppy.

I truly believe that each of us is mystified by the wonder of the creation of life and that we admire those human beings from whose bodies new life emerges. It's an epitome of creativity and accomplishment that I believe all males envy. Day after day I see a great deal of excitement when fathers are present at the birth of their children. It seems to me it's their deep respect for childbirth as the ultimate in the creative process. It's no accident that the phrase "That's my baby!" is one commonly used by men who have just finished a project or task for which they have a great sense of satisfaction and pride.

❦

Emotional Effects of Juvenile Diabetes

We've just discovered that our seventeen-year-old son is diabetic, and we know that the chances of his developing any number of problems that will shorten his life — from heart and circulatory afflictions to blindness and kidney disease — are greatly increased. Is a child who suffers such a serious disease going to be affected emotionally by his condition? How much should we talk about this with our son?

A child with diabetes is certainly affected emotionally, just as he would be affected by any condition that sets him apart from other children. Because he requires special medical care, he may be overprotected by his parents, given sympathy or ridicule by his peers, and feel envy and resentment from his siblings. And while he may not *want* to be singled out, it is true that greater vigilance on the part of his parents and teachers is necessary. The child soon becomes aware of this and in some cases uses the situation to manipulate adults, particularly if he has emotional problems or does not receive sufficient positive parental time and attention.

However, these emotional problems are secondary to the disease itself. The fact is that diabetes can affect a child's emotions directly. Basically, the treatment of diabetes requires daily injections of insulin, as well as a prescribed diet and exercise program. If these three elements are not properly balanced, a child can have physical and emotional reactions ranging from dizziness to confusion and crying, which are not only upsetting to the child but can obviously cause difficulties in school and on the playground and anxiousness for the parents.

I think it is most important for parents to be honest with their child about his condition. It is important for the diabetic child to know, for example, that if he is irritable and has trouble at school, it is not because he is "bad" or "stupid." Also, if parents try to hide the truth, the child is bound to lose trust in them when he finally learns about the illness. An informed child is much easier to treat and can make a better adjustment than the child who feels he is "different" from other children and does not know why. An honest and trusting relationship enables a child to ask his parents questions, which in turn allows the parents to give useful information while providing emotional support.

Most children want to know about the immediate implications of their illness and will not necessarily question the long-range implications. However, they understandably may wonder if their illness will cause them to die. While you would not want to go into medical statistics with young children, you can be sure that as they get older they will go to the library and read for themselves the available information on these matters. That is why I think it is fair to tell your son at this time that his is "a serious condition" that can cause him "to become very ill." You need not bring up all the facts concerning the possible kidney disease, circulatory afflictions, or blindness to which he is predisposed, but if he asks about such things specifically, let him know that people with diabetes can develop these problems if they don't take care of themselves. Explain further that "for this reason it is very important to take care of yourself and do the things the doctor tells you to."

A great deal of understanding and emotional support is necessary to help a child in such a situation.

❦

Preparing a Child for Hospitalization

Recently my neighbor's little girl was taken to the hospital with a broken arm. Aside from the shock and pain of the physical experience, she returned from the hospital depressed and frightened by her brief stay there — she says she hates hospitals and everyone in them. If my children ever have to go to the hospital, is there anything I can do to prevent this added trauma happening to them?

Children can be as fascinated by a hospital experience as they can be frightened by it. Generally speaking, it's appropriate for a child to be anxious and apprehensive about any unfamiliar situation, and hospitalization is no exception. In fact, the uncertainties and potentially uncomfortable or painful procedures a child undergoes in a hospital are built in to the experience itself. The more you can *eliminate* the uncertainties and provide emotional support for your child during the hospitalization, the less will be your child's anxiety. This means telling your child a few days before hospitalization why he is going to the hospital and what will be done. You must be realistic and descriptive of the situation as much as possible. This means you have to discuss, in detail, with your doctor the plans and procedures, and what pain and discomfort your child is likely to experience. It is frequently difficult for a parent to get this kind of detailed information, but, believe me, it's well worth it to put forth a great deal of effort even if you have to badger your doctor a little to get it. This applies not only to preparing your child for going into the hospital. Speak to the nurses as well as the doctors and ask them to keep you informed of what, when, where, and how things will be done to your child. In this way, you can help prepare your child during his hospital stay. In most hospitals for children, the nursing staff is very sensitive to the needs of children and is generally skillful in preparing children for procedures. Of course, there are exceptions. In general, the best hospitals for children usually include a recreation program or a "child-life" program. Hopefully, the nursing and recreational staffs of your child's hospital are affiliated with the Association for Child Care in Hospitals, which encourages such activities and conducts frequent meetings to sensitize and train child-care workers in hospitals with the emotional needs of children so that they are better equipped to have your child deal with the potential emotional stresses of hospital and medical care. I have been affiliated with this association for many years and am very proud of the work they are doing. Members of this association, in a sense, represent the child and are concerned not only with the child's emotional health but with his or her integrity and dignity.

Under no circumstances should you ever lie to your child about going into the hospital or what will take place there. The effects of misleading a child or lying to a child about medical or hospital procedures are devastating. Not only does it cause a child to lose trust in his parents, as well as all hospital personnel, but it causes a child to be angry, defiant, and resistant to any medical care. Children's resentment and distrust are understandable and very hard to correct after they have been lied to or misled even once. Moreover, it makes a child a difficult patient and one whose attitude about health care can become so negative that it can influence his or her pattern of health care throughout life. Adults who avoid regular medical check-ups or neglect important symptoms are frequently people who can trace their resentment toward the health-care profession to some of their early childhood experiences with doctors and hospitals.

For years I've seen children cope very effectively with uncomfortable and painful procedures when they've been told in advance what will happen. While they may cry and show some apprehensiveness, when it's over with they remember that you were honest and prepared them for what happened. This not only shows respect for their feelings but reinforces their trust in you. In addition, it gives a child an opportunity to mobilize his own resources for being able to cope with a stressful experience in a way that enhances the child's self-esteem. Feeling that he has come through an unpleasant procedure and done it with open awareness of what happened, the child has an opportunity to feel proud of himself. A child who has been misled or told, "This won't hurt a bit," and then it does, not only resents everyone involved but feels deceived and is deprived of his capacity for using his own resources in coping.

I feel very strongly about preparing children honestly for their hospital experiences and the parents' acceptance within the hospital to provide emotional support for the child. I've had innumerable children to treat and parents to consult with who suffered greatly for a long period of time as a result of even *one* poorly handled situation by health-care professionals. Hopefully, every hospital will have sufficient flexibility concerning visitation so that parents can be with their children when necessary to provide emotional support. Facilities should be available so that parents can stay overnight with their children when it's appropriate and can accompany children to many of the procedures that are potentially frightening to a child. As painless as an X ray may be, it is frequently very important for the parent to be present with the child because the setting and equipment are at times so austere and even frightening.

❧

Staying with the Hospitalized Child

My eight-year-old will be entering the hospital soon for a tonsillectomy. I have very firm feelings that I want to stay every moment with my little girl, and even stay all night — but my mother-in-law says that she didn't stay when her children had their tonsils out and that it isn't necessary. What are your feel-ings about this? Should parents of young children stay over-night with them? Do hospitals allow this now?

I believe that parents of children of any age should have the option of staying overnight with them when they are hos-pitalized. While it is not always necessary, at least the option should be open to them. Nighttime is frequently frightening to children, and this is particularly true if they are in a strange setting, suffering from pain and hearing noises and sounds around them from other patients who may be in discomfort. Adding to their fright may be the fact that different people take care of their needs at night than the people they have during the day. For this reason, the parent can offer continuity in care as well as the kind of emotional support that no one else in the life of the child can potentially provide. Some children, how-ever, prefer to "go it alone" at nighttime simply to show their independence and capacity to cope. Don't hesitate to speak to your child about this, and if she feels that you needn't stay overnight with her, by all means, accept her wishes. Many hospitals allow parents to stay overnight, but unfortunately many more do not. I believe it's sufficiently important for hos-pitals to allow parents to stay overnight with children that you should make every effort possible to find a hospital that does permit this.

❦

Children with Chronic Illness

My two-year-old granddaughter was recently diagnosed as hav-ing a serious blood disorder, and she will now have to go to the hospital for a number of tests. She's too little to understand much about this, and I wonder if she thinks she's being punished. Her five-year-old brother doesn't have to go to the hospital — could she think we love him more than her? Do you have any suggestions for us? Is there a way to convey to a very small child what is happening?

As hard as it may be to explain to a two-year-old what is happening, it's important to make the effort. So much communication between a parent and a child is through gesture and behavior that it's possible to provide a little child with protection and emotional security by staying with her as much as possible during tests. I have followed many children with serious blood diseases who have required frequent tests and transfusions and have adapted very well to them. The key to success lies in the hands of the hospital staff, as well as the emotional support and contact the parents can provide for the child. Nothing can be more painful for a child than a fear of abandonment, lack of regard for the child's feelings, or outright dishonesty. If your two-year-old granddaughter feels the emotional support from her parents, it is highly unlikely that she will interpret her experiences in the hospital as punishment. In no way would she feel that you love her less than her brother as long as a feeling of love is conveyed along with her medical care. Ironically, it is the sibling of the chronically handicapped child or the child with a prolonged illness who feels unloved and neglected because of the attention and parental time that is invested in the sick child.

❦

Child's Reaction to Parental Illness

I am rarely sick enough to stay in bed, but when I am, it seems to upset my children. I have two boys and a girl — their ages are six, nine, and eleven — and instead of helping around the house or bringing me juice or food, they become very distant and almost resentful of my condition. Are they angry with me because I'm ill? Am I being silly in thinking that they love me less when I'm sick? At all other times, they're very considerate and helpful. Why do they react this way when I'm sick?

I'm sure that your illness does not mean your children love you any less than they do when you're well. However, they may indeed be a little angry or annoyed with you because their "omnipotent" parent — who in their minds is capable of doing heroic things and able to take away discomfort — has become temporarily dependent and even somewhat helpless. Remember, being a little angry with someone doesn't necessarily detract from feelings of love. The fact that they are considerate and helpful at all other times tells me that they are probably irritable at the kind of role reversal your illness demands. Understandably, they prefer to have you available to meet their needs and maintain all the comforts of home and family to which they are so accustomed.

Even though your children seem to be ignoring your needs, you can be sure that underneath it all your illness causes a little anxiety. All children are fearful of losing parents and see illness as something that may take their parents away from them. This can cause some children to become very overprotective of their parents, hovering close by and not only catering to their every need but showing visible signs of their fear of loss. The fact that your children are doing quite the opposite does not mean that their fear of losing you is any less. Their method of dealing with their anxiety is to deny that you're ill in the first place. What they're saying, in a sense, is, "If we don't react to her as if she's ill, she's *not* ill — she's just being lazy." Seeing you as lazy causes them to either ignore your needs or show mild resentment. This reaction, incidentally, is not abnormal and should not be looked upon as insensitivity nor a lack of love or concern for your welfare.

I think you should approach the situation directly and explain that you don't feel well and need some help until you feel better. Let them know that you understand their resentment toward you for not being available to run things the way you usually do. Nevertheless, you need them to help around the house and bring juice and food. Don't hesitate to tell them that you *really* feel sick and that you're not simply trying to get them to wait on you. Remind them that when they were ill, it felt good to have someone take care of them and do little things that made it easier until they were well again.

❦

Explaining Chronic Parental Illness

My husband has been very active all his life. We've just found out that he has multiple sclerosis, and we know this will cause many changes in his life and the lives of all of us within the family. Needless to say, we're all very upset and want to know what the best approach is in dealing with this problem. What should we tell other people when they ask about MS, and how should we handle our children's reactions?

Basically, MS is a disease of the central nervous system, and people with MS do not usually feel pain because of their condition. Doctors do not yet know what causes it, and while there is no cure, there are methods of treatment and medication that are helpful.

The main symptoms that occur are dizziness, weakness, problems with vision, lack of coordination, muscle stiffness, and in more severe cases, paralysis of the arms and legs. The symptoms of the disease come and go; they sometimes fade away for long periods of time. Let your friends know that multiple sclerosis is *not* contagious, is not hereditary, and is not a fatal disease.

A person with MS is more susceptible to other diseases, such as respiratory or urinary infections, and needs to take greater care when it comes to matters of diet, exercise, and rest. Point out that a person with MS can live a full and productive life. In fact, two out of three people with MS are still able to walk twenty-five years after they are diagnosed.

Unquestionably, everyone within the family will have to make adjustments as MS progresses. I'm sure when you first heard of your husband's diagnosis, it made you very depressed and upset. That is perfectly normal. It's important that you help your children understand that your husband has an illness. Don't try to hide it because children are very perceptive and sensitive and will only lose trust in you if they feel that you are hiding some truth from them. At the same time, it's not necessary to go into all the details of what MS is. It's important for them to know that their father may have to take less of an active part in physical activities and may not be able to do some of the things he was able to do before. Nevertheless, it's important to point out that in no way will it affect his love for them.

❦

Childhood Depression

Over the last several months our five-year-old boy has seemed constantly withdrawn, unhappy, and tearful. My husband thinks I should just let him alone, or try to jolly him out of it. But I can't help worrying — is it possible for young children to suffer from depression the way adults do?

The kinds of depression that can afflict adults fall into three general categories. Reactive depression occurs in response to real happenings in one's life. The death of a loved one, a family breakup, the loss of a job, the move to a new home — all these can cause a person to feel grief or fear or sadness, which is perfectly understandable under the circumstances. Usually, these feelings pass with time, but if they are unresolved or repressed, they may settle into a more lasting depression that could require professional treatment.

Endogenous depression is due to an actual physical disorder or chemical imbalance within a person's body. It sometimes may be periodic and relate to changes such as menstruation, menopause, or other physical or organic disturbances that occur from time to time.

The third kind of depression, neurotic depression, is basically caused by inner and deeply rooted conflicts, which in a sense weaken a person's capacity to deal with the normal problems of everyday life.

Children rarely suffer from neurotic depression. It is sometimes possible, however, for them to suffer endogenous depression — on rare occasions they do have emotional reactions that are due to physical factors. Poor nutrition, a chemical imbalance, or even a hormonal imbalance can affect a child's mood and behavior, so don't hesitate to discuss the possibility of this with your pediatrician.

But when children are in an emotional state such as the one you describe, they most likely are reacting to the circumstances in their lives. Something is making your son feel unhappy and helpless. No, you should not try to "jolly" him out of it or just "let him alone." Examine what's happening in his life to see if you can uncover the reasons for his upset. He may be feeling rejected or unloved, or he may be feeling a sense of loss. Some children are able to verbalize the reasons for their unhappiness to their parents, while others require some professional help to find out what the underlying causes are. But whether he talks to you of his own accord or the help of a counselor or therapist is necessary, your child is clearly depressed and should be helped.

For families of every age, depression should be taken very seriously. It can lead to morbid feelings of helplessness and at times an overwhelming inability to cope. In certain cases it may even lead to suicide.

❦

Children and Household Chores

Our daughters are ages thirteen, nine, and seven. We have given each of them certain household chores to do every day, such as washing dishes, setting the table, and helping with housework. But lately they've been saying I give them too much to do, and they don't have time to play or be with their friends. Do you think they're too young to handle these chores? Are they right when they say that I'm asking too much of them?

No, I don't think they are too young to handle these chores, but they may be right when they say that you are asking too much of them. I think it's important for children to share in family responsibilities to develop a sense of their own capabilities, as well as to gain a feeling of importance within the family unit. If, however, these tasks begin to interfere with other things that your growing daughters feel are also important, you may have to reassess the situation. Perhaps they are moving into a stage of development where their need to be with friends is greater.

I suggest you discuss the situation with them openly and frankly. You should respect their feelings and look upon their dissatisfaction seriously. Let them know you don't want to "exploit" them or burden them unfairly; at the same time, everyone in the family has a role to play in the maintenance of their home. Find out what alternatives your daughters would suggest, and try to work out some compromise situation. You might be surprised to find that the modifications they suggest are reasonable and acceptable to you.

It's very important for parents to be flexible and open-minded enough to consider the suggestions of their children and to accept alternative and reasonable ideas that they present. In this way, children not only develop a capacity to compromise but also learn that parents can be understanding people who respect their feelings and can be dealt with rationally. If you take a hard and fast line and refuse to listen or compromise, the so-called generation gap could become a substantial wedge between you and your children.

❦

Teaching Children to Share

What do you feel is the best way to teach children how to share? I have four children — two teenagers and two in grade school — and there's definitely an "every man for himself" attitude in our house. I'd like them to share responsibilities and chores and to care for one another so that we'd be more of a team, but I don't know how to bring this about.

I think that we as parents often tend to forget how important it is for children to learn to care for others, and the best place to teach this is in the home. A responsive parent who instills in a child a sense of responsible and loving concern for others makes an invaluable imprint on a young personality. The personal satisfaction it can give your child when he or she helps you, a brother or sister, or a friend or neighbor is one of life's greatest rewards. And, of course, from a practical standpoint, many homes could not function comfortably without the care and assistance of the younger members of the family.

Unquestionably, older siblings can and should be expected to help out with younger ones. But to ensure that this is a positive experience for everyone involved, it is up to parents to conscientiously evaluate each situation and the maturity of the children involved.

A key factor is the parents' attitude — and the appreciation they express to their children about this experience. Parents are sometimes quick to *demand* that an older child care for a younger sibling simply as an obligation; in doing so, they show little or no positive recognition for what the older child has done. This can lead to resentment and a resistance to sharing all family responsibilities. By openly discussing with your children your reasons for needing their help, and by showing your pride and gratitude for their efforts and energy, you will give your children a feeling of self-esteem, as well as show your respect for their feelings.

It is also important to remember that children have a right to live their own lives, and that while family responsibilities are important, they should not be so extensive that they greatly limit the older children's participation in activities with their peers. Being constantly burdened with caring for a little brother or sister, while all the other children are socializing or playing without such encumbrances, can understandably cause resentment toward parents, as well as toward the little ones.

As far as other general guidelines are concerned, it is best to avoid having one child assume responsibility for another child who is close in age — say, less than three or four years apart. Such children are likely to be at similar stages of development; they are not separated by a time span that makes one clearly more knowledgeable or reliable than the other. (It can be a good idea, however, for children of similar ages to mutually "watch out" for each other in day-to-day situations — and to be alert if the other gets into trouble or needs help.)

For children who are more separated in years, the age and maturity of each are the factors to consider, as well as the time span that they are to be left together. Although younger children can "keep an eye on" an infant or toddler under the parents' supervision, for instance, such a small child should not be left completely in the trust of a youngster of eight or nine, whereas a young teenager is quite capable of watching an infant for an evening.

The personalities and characteristics of all the children involved are of course also important. The older child should have sufficiently good judgment and a sound capacity for evaluating and anticipating danger. The younger should have a reasonable sense of trust in the older's authority — and should be a child who is emotionally stable and free from any particular problems of temperament and health. Placing an impulsive or hyperactive child in the care of an older child, for instance, can be potentially hazardous to both. Even adults have difficulty handling children who are constantly racing about or into mischief, and asking an older sibling to take on this responsibility can cause real tension. And if the envy, jealousy, or rivalry between two children is intense, you can be sure that leaving one in the care of the other will lead to "war" between the two. Some children exercise authority over a younger sibling in a way that is hostile or tends to terrorize the younger child. And under no circumstances should you ever force an older child to care for a younger sibling as a punishment for past misbehavior. Clearly this could cause real resentment and even retaliation against the younger child. Remember that in the long run, leaving immature or squabbling children together can *cause* you more problems than it will ever solve.

The situations in which children are left together are important also. Under no circumstances should a child of perhaps ten, eleven, or twelve years of age assume responsibility for a younger child near a pool or any other body of water where a drowning can occur. If things go wrong, in all fairness you cannot blame the older child. In my years of practice as a psychologist I have encountered some tragic occurrences, which, although purely accidental, left permanent scars on an older sibling whose younger charge was severely injured or died during their time together. The specific episodes I have in mind involve a child's drowning, a death by fire, and a youngster who was hit by an automobile. Totally apart from the tragedy itself, the older child was left with a residue of guilt and remorse.

In my experience, the more positive recognition that parents show toward older siblings who assume any of these responsibilities, the more the youngsters naturally take these responsibilities upon themselves. Ultimately they will need little or no prompting to help out. Some children I know take over quite spontaneously in helping younger siblings with homework, listening to their problems, and even giving advice and offering to take them to school. Other children I know take great pride in teaching a younger child to ride a bicycle, and enjoy the experience of sharing a movie. And younger siblings, aware of the recognition that an older brother or sister gets in caring for them, will look forward to the day when they themselves can care for other children.

My own son, Eric, has always volunteered to do things with his sister, Pia, who is six years younger. Eric, who baby-sat for others as a means of earning extra money, marveled at his sister's lovely paintings and unhesitatingly helped her with some of her science projects at school. I have always been pleased with his sensitivity to his younger sister and admired the hours he spent observing her as an infant and young baby. I am sure the pride I have expressed in his warmth and patience with his sister have helped make this a positive experience for him — and the charm and love that radiates from Pia clearly indicates that she feels the same way.

Pia, in turn, has picked up Eric's concern for younger children. She badgers me constantly to invite people to dinner who have babies so that she can take care of them while their parents are eating. She is always proud to be asked to come and play with a neighbor's young child to free the parent to do something else.

Sharing responsibilities within a family unit leads to a greater sense of self-esteem for all, serves to reinforce family ties, and provides children with a positive model regarding human life. I believe the greatest satisfactions human beings can gain in life are those that involve the sharing of some of life's burdens and the deep sense of fulfillment that results.

❦

Paying Children for Family Chores

Instead of giving an allowance to our children every week, my husband pays them for specific chores they do around the house. Is this right, or should children have a set amount of money that they can count on receiving? And should an allowance be withheld if a child has misbehaved?

Children should indeed have money that is their own and that is not dependent upon anything else, other than perhaps a change in the family's financial status. But it's as inappropriate for you to pay a child for individual chores as it would be for each member of the family to pay you at the end of a meal. A child who is paid for completing individual tasks will not develop a feeling that his or her efforts are an integral part of the overall effort needed to keep the family going. It's not important to establish whose contributions are the most essential, just that everyone does a share.

Also, it's important for children to know that they can count on receiving a set amount of money, paid to them regularly, because it gives them the opportunity to plan ahead for purchases, and perhaps even to learn how to save their money by putting part of each allowance into the bank.

Parents who withhold all or part of a child's allowance as punishment for misbehavior often get fast, positive results. However, I believe that the long-term losses resulting from this kind of punishment are more significant than the immediate benefits. By withholding allowances for misbehavior, or giving financial bonuses for "good" behavior, the child begins to associate money with love and acceptance, and I don't believe money should be used in this way. It's far more effective in the long run if the punishment is directly related to the rules that have been violated.

❦

The Clumsy Child

My eight-year-old daughter just goes barreling into everything, making a mess that others are left to lament or clean up. The other day she came home from school in great excitement and ricocheted into a family heirloom vase and sent it crashing to the floor. On other occasions she says she wants to "help" — in cooking, changing the litter box, whatever — but she makes such a mess that I end up being cross with her. These "mad bomber" tendencies are really getting on my nerves. I know she's not doing this on purpose, and I don't want to squelch her spirited nature — but I also think she should have some responsibility for her actions. What should I say to her?

I don't think you should discourage her enthusiasm for wanting to help around the house. You are very fortunate that she feels this way, and it is now your task to help her develop the skills involved in the tasks she undertakes. By being severely critical of her actions and losing patience with her, you run a real risk of squelching her spirit — and also of discouraging her from wanting to help when she is older.

As far as family heirlooms are concerned, perhaps you ought to put these items and other such valuables in a more secure place until her clumsiness subsides. In addition, you should assist her for a while in her efforts in cooking, changing the litter box, and any other tasks she wants to engage in, and show in a *positive* way how she can do these things carefully and without accidents. Basically, people learn by their mistakes — if there is someone to guide them and show them alternative ways of doing things that will bring them greater success and satisfaction. If you show pride in your daughter's gradual accomplishments in these tasks, she will not only master them but move on to do others successfully as well.

❦

Explaining Alcoholism to Children

How old do children have to be before they can understand about alcoholism? My children are four and seven — and they love their grandfather. But for the last year he's had a terrible drinking problem, and even though no one has ever talked openly to them about it, it seems to me that the children must notice when their grandfather slurs his words and stumbles around. Should I try to explain the situation to them? Do you think they notice and understand what's happening?

It's time to explain about alcoholism when children start asking questions — and children who are directly exposed to someone with a drinking problem will probably ask these questions at an earlier age. Your children are certainly old enough to notice what is going on and should have some kind of explanation for what they see. Children of four and seven are able to understand that different people have different kinds of sicknesses. Explain that some people drink too much because they are unhappy about themselves, that they may start out drinking very little just to relax, but as time goes on, they need to drink more and more. Then they can't seem to stop themselves, even though they realize that drinking so much can be very harmful to them. Tell them that this is why Grandpa slurs his words and stumbles around from time to time. Explain that when people drink a lot, it makes them feel strange and do strange things. Let them know some of the hazards that can occur when a person is drunk — that people who drink too much can be dangerous when they drive or may become so uncoordinated that they may injure themselves or others. While this may frighten your children somewhat, it will help them understand the consequences of behavior that occurs when a person is unable to control his or her impulses. I think it's fair to add that many people drink occasionally when they celebrate special events, or before mealtimes at the end of a hard day, because it makes them feel happier and more relaxed. Emphasize the fact that people who drink a lot, and have become alcoholics, are not necessarily bad people but merely people who require understanding and help so that they can overcome their problems.

Treat your children's questions with respect, and make sure

that their curiosity is satisfied. In this way you will be helping them understand their grandfather's problems while giving them valuable knowledge to guard against their getting caught up in such a problem themselves later on.

❦

Problems with Older Relatives

I have an elderly aunt who lives in a nursing home in the area, and every year I invite her to come for Christmas. My family grumbles a lot about this — and it is true that she's difficult, obstinate, and childish — but she has no other family and nowhere else to go. Am I selfish to insist on inviting her, even though the others object? What arguments can I use to convince my family?

I don't think you are at all "selfish" in inviting her, and I see every reason in the world for including her in your celebrations. It takes little imagination to understand the loneliness of being in an institution far away from family and friends at such a time. Ask your family how *they* would feel in the same situation. After you have talked out this problem, they should be better able to handle your aunt with understanding, patience, and goodwill.

❦

The Overly Critical Child

Within the last several months, my eight-year-old has taken to insulting me. She'll constantly say things like "Mommy, you talk funny" and "You're not as pretty as the other mommies" and "You're stupid." The other day I snapped back that there were things wrong with her, too — and she burst into tears because I'd said "something mean" to her. Why is she verbalizing all this criticism? And how should I handle it?

Children learn a great deal about coping with life's problems from their parents. In fact, I've always felt that children whose parents have had family problems and coped with them effectively have more resources available themselves for dealing with similar problems if they arise later on in their own lives.

It sounds to me as if your daughter is presenting you with some specific issues that she herself needs help with. As you know, children are often very direct in their remarks and sometimes hurt one another's feelings. When this happens, they often don't know what to do. I think your daughter is saying things to you that she may have said to other people or that other people have said to her, and she simply doesn't know how to deal with these comments or the situations in which they arise. She's obviously sensitive about these things, or she would not have burst into tears when you replied to her in kind. In a sense, she wants to see your reactions to these "insulting" remarks. If you could respond without losing your "cool," maintaining your self-esteem and avoiding going on the defensive or offensive yourself, you would be providing your child with the tools for handling these same remarks if they are made to her. When she says, "You are not as pretty as other mommies," just say, "I'm sure some mommies are prettier than I am and some are not. What counts more than how pretty you are is what kind of person you are." To a remark such as, "You're stupid," you might reply that "there are many things people know and many things they don't know, and it doesn't mean a person is stupid if they don't have all the answers to everything." By delving more into her remarks while maintaining your composure and integrity, you can help your daughter develop the skills for handling other people's criticisms.

❦

Being Affectionate

The other day my eight-year-old niece said in a very hurt voice that she thought I didn't love her because I never kissed and hugged her. I love her very dearly, but it's true that I'm not particularly demonstrative with her. Should I do more squeezing and cuddling?

Tell your niece what you've just told me. Let her know that you do indeed love her; explain that different people express their love in different ways, and some are more demonstrative than others. You might want to add that some people are very demonstrative but not necessarily very sincere — but be careful not to press this point so as to confuse her at this time.

Children are generally very sensitive to people's reactions and can tell how people really feel about them. It's possible that your niece may have sensed you were preoccupied with something else, and this was her way of saying that she wanted a little more recognition from you. Most children get their ideas about affection from their parents, and your niece obviously associates affectionate gestures with real love. Because of this, you may want to be more generous with your cuddles and squeezes — after all, you're lucky to have a little niece who not only enjoys such gestures but tells you so. She obviously cares about your feelings for her; surely she deserves those extra hugs.

Teenager Handling Parental Arguments

I'm a high school student and the only one of three children living at home. My problem is that I've become a go-between in my parents' petty arguments. They often consult me to decide who's "right," and each one expects me to support his or her "side" of the disagreement. Why do my parents do this? How should I handle this situation?

It must be excruciating for you to deal with your feelings in a situation such as this. After all, your parents should protect you from this kind of discomfort rather than cause it to happen in the first place.

When your parents ask you to take sides, each is using you as a weapon. Your mother and father must obviously feel desperate and need support, but you didn't cause their problems, and it is certainly not your responsibility to solve them.

There is no easy way for you to handle this situation. If you try to avoid expressing your own feelings and take a passive role in which you say or do nothing, your own internal tensions can build to cause you undue emotional stress as well as physical symptoms. On the other hand, "taking sides" can cause you to feel a sense of guilt and a fear of rejection from the parent with whom you do not side.

I believe you should tell your parents in no uncertain terms that their disagreements are their *own*. Let them know — both individually and together — that you do not want to hear about their problems and that you have no intention of taking sides in their disagreements. Do not hesitate to let them know you are not only unhappy about this but actually angry about being placed in such a position. There is no easy way out of this situation, but hiding your own feelings is not the solution.

If at all possible, you should find some friend, relative, or professional in whom you have some confidence and trust and to whom you can tell your problems. At least, find some relief by sharing the agony this situation creates for you.

Adult Fear of Cancer

My husband claims that cancer can be hereditary, and while I do not believe this, I worry that he believes it. My husband's father was stricken with cancer, as was his uncle, and now my husband seems to just take it for granted that he too will be afflicted. He talks pessimistically —and quite frequently — about this happening. If he continues to talk like this, do you think it might turn out to be a self-fulfilling prophecy? He is fifty-five and, as far as we know, in good health.

Studies have shown that there is something called *somatic compliance*, in which the body seems to adapt itself physically to a person's psychological wishes. While this phenomenon is certainly more complicated than a simple "self-fulfilling prophecy," it is true that continued emotional stress can cause real physical problems. It is also true that in some cases there may be a hereditary predisposition to certain conditions or diseases such as cancer, but this certainly does not mean that everyone in the same family line will ultimately develop that condition. So while your husband's anxiety is not altogether unfounded, it is also obviously out of proportion to the reality of his own situation.

Anyone who is deeply concerned and preoccupied with a situation that does not really exist has a psychological problem. Every time your husband raises this issue, refer him to his doctor for an expert opinion. Perhaps you should also tactfully suggest that he see a certified psychologist or psychiatrist to help him deal with his anxiety — or you might talk with his doctor or clergyman about broaching the subject to him. Make it clear to your husband that you have no doubts about his "stability" but that you think it might help him if he discusses his anxiety with an outside professional who is not part of his everyday life.

Handling Hero Worship of the Wrong Person

Our son is twelve — and he idolizes his uncle, a sweet but kind of dopey boy of twenty-two who envisions himself a "swinger" and works as a drummer in a rock band. We're fond of our twenty-two-year-old relative, but he's really quite aimless about his life and has attitudes and values that my husband and I do do not wish our son to adopt. Should we intervene in this situation?

I've known many youngsters who develop this sort of hero worship toward an older boy or girl whose lifestyle is so different from their own. This adulation is usually transitory, and there is no reason to assume that your son will adopt the same attitudes and values as his uncle, even though he might tend to imitate him in some ways.

I do believe, however, that it's important for parents to express their own views and values to their children, letting them know the kind of behavior of which they approve or disapprove. While you should not be dogmatic or harsh in the expression of these attitudes, it's important to let your children know that you live by certain standards — and give them your reasons for believing in such principles. At the same time, I don't think it's wise for parents to flatly impose these values on their children. Such rigidity can cause defiance and rebelliousness toward the values that parents hold dear or, conversely, can result in a blind compliance based on a fear of punishment or loss of love. If your children feel that you love them no matter what — even though at times you may disapprove of their specific behavior — they should be open in discussing their feelings with you. This kind of relationship gives children the independence to develop their own standards of behavior by choice rather than coercion, and in all likelihood their values will then be drawn from those within their own family.

In this particular case, I don't think you ought to intervene in your son's relationship with his uncle, a relationship that sounds gratifying for both of them. But, continuing to indicate your fondness for your relative, also point out to your son that you have reservations about the way the older boy has organized his life. By talking to him openly in this way, your child will feel that he is a significant and esteemed member of your family, and he should be far more influenced by your lifestyle than that of his uncle.

❦

Responsible Handling of Accidents

Recently my husband and our two sons, ages twelve and nine, were driving home and came upon the scene of an automobile accident. We slowed down, saw that there were plenty of people on hand to help, and continued on our way rather than add to the congestion at the scene. Both of our sons later questioned why we hadn't stopped, and we explained that we would have pulled over if we thought we could have done something to help. Later I worried that our children had lost respect for us. Did we do the right thing?

You dealt with the situation perfectly. Nothing can cause more confusion at the scene of an accident than a crowd of gawking people, and a traffic jam of curiosity seekers only interferes with police and ambulance access. Your explanation to your children was clear and rational, and I can't believe that they would lose respect for you.

Your children's desire to help is commendable and certainly reflects the kind of values you have obviously conveyed to them.

But the experience you have just described should be equally edifying: It shows them that it's as important to avoid contributing to confusion and chaos as it is to offer help when it's really necessary.

❦

Visiting Elderly at Nursing Home

My father is very elderly and in a nursing home, in such poor health that doctors advise us not to bring him home for Christmas. Last year I bundled up our children, ages six and nine, to visit him on Christmas day, something they did with great reluctance. This year when I announced we had to go again, the children were vocal about their unhappiness — my son even wailed, "Mommy, that will ruin our Christmas day!" Am I wrong to insist that my children do this?

I believe you are absolutely correct in feeling you should make this visit with your children. I can understand their reaction: Many nursing homes are in fact depressing places, which is all the more reason why all of you should visit your father. It would brighten up his life and bring him closer to his family. (And frankly speaking, visits to your father should not be limited to holidays.)

As far as "ruining" Christmas, now is the time for you to have a discussion with your children about the importance of Christmas as a *family* holiday, and the roles each of them plays within that framework. Make it clear to your children that they have real responsibilities for the feelings of those close to them and that their grandfather is still part of their family, even though his health is very poor. Emphasize the fact that he is *your* parent and that your feelings for him are much like your children's feelings for you. I also would point out that someday you yourself could be ill and would certainly want your children and grandchildren to continue to include you in their lives. Explain that at times we may have to do things that are not pleasant but must be done, nevertheless, simply out of a sense of responsibility.

Life would be better for everyone if we could teach our children that there is satisfaction — real satisfaction — in bringing joy and happiness into the lives of other people, even if it means going out of our way at times or subjecting ourselves to situations that we might avoid otherwise. If you can get this idea across to your children, you will have given them the greatest Christmas gift of all.

❧

Child Abuse

Lately I read more and more about child abuse, and I find it both shocking and incomprehensible. What's going on in the minds of the parents who do such a thing? If they hate children so much, why do they have them in the first place? And why don't the children involved tell their teachers or other adults what's happening and ask for help?

In my experience, most parents who are child abusers don't really hate children. For the most part, they are people who have poor control over their impulses, and when frustrated, they become overwhelmed and lash out in destructive ways against those who are closest to them and often the most defenseless. Many of these people have grown up in homes that were lacking in love and consistent discipline, and many were beaten as children themselves. They failed to learn how to come to terms with their own anger and aggression. For instance, I've known many young mothers — particularly unwed mothers — who have tried to make up for the lack of love in their own lives by having a baby that they hoped would love *them*, and give them a feeling of being important. Needless to say, instead of providing such parents with a sense of emotional gratification, children make even greater demands upon them. The frustration that ensues, in conjunction with the inability to cope with such feelings, frequently sparks the outbursts of rage that lead to child abuse.

Such problems are of course in no way limited to unwed mothers. They exist at all levels in our society, for both men and women. We grow up in an atmosphere that tolerates and even condones violence, and that often sanctions physical punishment as a way of getting children to behave. I am appalled at the amount of institutional child abuse that exists in our society, and was very distressed when the Supreme Court sanctioned paddling in schools. This sort of disrespect for the fundamental human rights of children serves as a foundation for child abuse; it goes hand in hand with the benign neglect of children that I feel is so prevalent in families today. Parents feel justified, and are in many ways encouraged, in spending more and more time away from their children. They spend more time at the office or go off to "do their own thing." In my opinion, this contributes to the slighting of the emotional needs of children during those crucial years when the foundation for their future personality is being formed. In addition to creating a climate that denigrates the needs and rights of children, many people have unfortunately not been adequately and realistically prepared for the responsibilities of parenthood, and their disappointment and discouragement mounts as they encounter the normal problems of everyday life with their children.

Some children whose parents have abused them *do* tell other people, but many don't out of fear of parental revenge. Moreover, most children who have been abused still prefer being with their parents to what might happen if they were taken away from them.

There is no doubt in my mind that something must be done to protect our children from the deplorable child abuse we read about. In addition to reeducating society about how and why situations like this occur, people must be willing to get involved if they suspect such abuse is happening. While there may be variations from area to area, every state has some facility for dealing with these matters, and it's possible to report instances of child abuse without giving your own identity. If you have real reason to suspect a child is is being battered, ask your local telephone operator for a listing of child-protection services in your area — or there may be a hotline listing that you can call. Also, a clergyman or a member of your local police department or social service agency should be able to give you guidance about whom to contact. At the same time, I think we must show the same concern about emotional neglect or abuse, which can be even more damaging to children in the long run but which seems to less of a dramatic event and so gets less attention from the press and politicians.

❧

Thumb Sucking

What is the best way to stop thumb sucking? My mother says to put iodine or some other bitter material on my son's thumb, but I'm not sure this is right. How do you break a young child of this habit — or is it a habit that should be broken?

I am totally against putting iodine or any bitter material on a child's thumb to stop sucking. Most children give up the habit of thumb sucking by the time they reach five and then limit their thumb sucking to bedtime and periods of stress. Making an issue of thumb sucking can make the problem worse, but above all, it can magnify the issue out of proportion and create a situation where parent and child are pitted against each other unnecessarily.

If parents tease children, or nag them about the habit, it tends to undermine the child's self-confidence. I am inclined to let the child alone and allow the habit to dissipate of its own accord. I know there are dangers of dental deformities, and most dentists are deeply concerned about this problem. But my own experience in dealing with children whose parents took a firm or punitive position on thumb sucking tells me that it is easier to correct any dental deformities that might occur than it is to deal with the emotional problems caused by parental obsession over the matter.

❦

Mental Deterioration of Elderly Relatives

We have an elderly aunt in our family who is beloved by all our children, and who has participated in many activities and "adventures" with them. But lately our aunt's physical and mental health has begun to deteriorate, and we can see that our children are puzzled by this change in her. Should we try to explain to our children what is happening? Should we try to discourage them from seeing so much of her now?

On the contrary, you should encourage them to see *more* of her now. That way, the changes your children see in your aunt will seem less traumatic, and they will learn important lessons about dealing with such changes in those they love.

As far as your aunt herself is concerned, frequent visits by the children will probably improve her morale and give her a greater feeling of vitality as she continues to maintain the loving relationship she has had with your children all along. I firmly believe that as a person's mental outlook improves, so does his or her physical health. Making life more meaningful and enjoyable for your aunt can possibly serve to arrest — and perhaps even reverse — her failing health.

As far as explaining to your children what is happening, I believe that you should be direct and open with them about your aunt's condition. Give them the opportunity of asking anything they want to know about how she is, what has caused her condition, and what the future may bring. Reply to their questions as honestly as you can, and do not hesitate to tell them that you too "don't know" some of the answers to everything. The respect and honesty you show in dealing with them, and your willingness to help them come to terms with life's realities (and getting old is certainly an important one of them), are things they will remember and value throughout their lives.

❦

The Loveless Marriage

My marriage is an unhappy one, yet because of financial difficulties, my husband and I often talk about divorce but never really follow through on it. Our children are ages eight and twelve, and I can't help wondering — will this loveless atmosphere between my husband and myself affect them?

Under these circumstances your children will be living in an environment in which they see little or no affection between their parents, and this is bound to set for them a distorted example of what a marital relationship should be like. If there is prolonged tension and discomfort, your children also may begin to seek the emotional satisfaction they need elsewhere — outside the home.

There is much to be said for a couple who tries to make a marriage work and continues to live together in an attempt to do so; I believe that every effort should be made to work out marital problems before actually going through with a divorce. In your case, things seem to have deteriorated badly. While no direct harm will come to your children by living in this unhappy atmosphere, there are bound to be subtle negative effects. It is important for you and your husband to treat each other with courtesy and respect during this time — and to make it clear to your children that your collective and individual love for them remains strong and undiminished.

❦

Breaking Promises to Children

My husband is always promising things that he ultimately cannot follow through on. I worry about this, especially where our children are concerned. He tells them he'll buy them motorbikes or take them away on a camping trip — and he means what he says when he says it — but somehow these plans and promises rarely materialize and then the children are puzzled and disappointed. Am I right in thinking this is a serious problem, or is it nothing to worry about? I don't want to undermine my husband in front of the children, but I feel that I should speak up when he's rhapsodizing about all the things he says he's going to do or buy for them — and never does.

I believe you are absolutely right in considering this a serious problem. Children understandably lose confidence in parents who make promises and don't follow through. What is most disheartening to them is not the motorbikes or vacations that never materialize, but the fact that they can't depend on what their parents say. Their mistrust breeds unhappy consequences: Children begin to ignore parental guidance or advice, question the sincerity of emotional support or reassurance their parents give during periods or stress or turmoil, and even wonder if they are truly loved.

I think you should discuss very seriously with your husband the possible consequences of his failure to deliver on what he promises. Perhaps you can help him work out the plans to make his ideas come true. Don't undermine him in front of your children. Instead, you might "tone down" some of his promises at the time they are being made, altering them into more practical ideas in the hope that he *will* follow through. For example, if he promises a camping vacation, you might suggest that if a camping trip doesn't work out, you can all spend a few days together at a favorite spot that is fairly accessible. In effect, you'll be telling your children, "Dad is generous and sincere about his promises, but it's sometimes hard to make them *all* come true. If this plan doesn't work out, something else will." This at least provides a greater possibility for the realization of some plan that your children will enjoy, while it puts their father's promises into a perspective that they will be better able to deal with.

❦

The Undisciplined Child

My sister's husband died several years ago, and she's raised their eight-year-old boy by herself. The problem is that the child is very undisciplined and rowdy. The other night he burst into one of his typical tantrums in a restaurant, and his mother barely did anything to quiet him. My husband and I are our nephew's only other family, and we feel a responsibility for the child's upbringing. Yet we hesitate to correct his deportment when his mother is right there, and seemingly untroubled by it. What should we do?

I think you should not interfere directly with your sister's handling of her child. It would not only be confusing for the child to deal with two different sources of authority but might arouse resentment on your sister's part toward you. It could also undermine your sister's position with her child and make a bad situation even worse.

I suggest you pick a time when you and your sister are by yourselves and comfortable in conversation together, and feel free to discuss serious matters openly and in a nonthreatening way. Talk with your sister about how she feels about raising her child alone. Give her an opportunity to express her feelings. You might find that she very much wants your help, and at that time it would be appropriate to offer it You might point out that you have noticed how difficult it is for her to handle her son in some situations — and from her reactions you can gauge her ability to accept your suggestions for her child's behavior. At that time you can tactfully explain to her how much children need firm consistency in the establishment of rules and regulations.

This approach can bring you and your sister closer together and would offer the help you feel she needs. But by jumping into the situation directly and reprimanding the child in a public place, I am afraid you might create even more emotional tension that would do nothing to help the situation and might do much to hurt it.

❦

Career Mother vs. Housemaker – Stepmother

My ex-husband has remarried, and his wife bakes bread and sews curtains and spends a lot of time making her home attractive. I have not remarried and am now working — and I am excited about developing my career. The problem is with my ten-year-old daughter and eight-year-old son: They love their new stepmother and talk about all the wonderful cookies she bakes and the patches she sews on their dungarees, things I wouldn't be interested in doing even if I did have the time. I want my kids to think I'm terrific, too. Should I force myself to bake and sew even though I have no interest in doing so?

Your feelings are perfectly understandable. In a sense, you feel your children's admiration of their stepmother is a threat to your relationship with them. But you must avoid at all costs becoming competitive with her. If you turn this into a problem, your children will suffer; they will be torn by feelings of disloyalty and guilt instead of being free to enjoy the best of what both parents have to offer.

At this time, it may be hard for your children to share the newly found excitement you feel in your work because they have no knowledge of or contact with it. However, if you have them visit the place you work, meet the people you enjoy working with, and discuss with them the things you are doing, I am sure they will eventually speak to their stepmother with as much pride in *your* activities as they speak to you about hers.

No, I don't think you should force yourself to bake and sew. You would not only be doing something you resent but would be setting up a challenge situation that would serve no useful purpose whatsoever. Be yourself and try to share in your children's pleasure. This will eventually make them willing and eager to share in yours.

Responsibility for the Messy Room

Although I have begged my twelve-year-old son to keep his room clean, he does nothing about it. Finally, I went in one day, scooped up armsful of old magazines and papers — and even socks and toys — and heaved it all out in the garbage. This has caused a huge commotion in our house. My son seems to feel his room is utterly off-limits, and he can do as he pleases in it. But I feel it's up to him to keep it clean — and if he doesn't, I can throw out what I want. Was I wrong to do what I did? Is a child's room his own domain? How can we work this out?

His room cannot be utterly "off-limits" to you because it's your responsibility to maintain your home. However, this doesn't mean that you should have free access at all times. You must show regard for your son's feelings and possessions. I can understand your frustration about the accumulation of things that you feel are useless; nonetheless, they may be important to *him.*

Apologize to your son for having to resort to such drastic measures, but explain that you finally became so frustrated that you simply felt compelled to take some kind of action. Let him know that you want him to have his privacy and the right to surround himself with his own belongings but that his untidiness makes you very unhappy, and you must have his help in solving the problem. Don't set up this confrontation as a win-or-lose situation where one of you is bound to lose face, but think of it as a cooperative endeavor that involves compromise on both sides.

In such situations, which arouse intense emotions, it's best to work out solutions, not at the moment of crisis, but when all seems well and communication is at its best. Don't hesitate to say, "I love you very much, you're a wonderful child — I only wish you could help me work out a solution to a problem that interferes with our having happiness and satisfaction more of the time." By appealing to him in this way, you not only take constructive steps toward a solution but help him understand that human beings can get frustrated — and that even parents sometimes need the help of their children in resolving human problems.

❧

Respecting a Child's Personal Life

My children get very upset if I, in their presence, tell others about something they've told me about schoolwork or their friends or activities. Then if I stop and tell my son or daughter to go on with the story, that just seems to make things worse — and they refuse to say anything. What's the problem? Do they want to tell their own stories? Or do they want no one to tell those stories?

Most sensitive children react angrily when an adult reveals personal information about them without first asking their permission to do so. Your children have told you alone what's going on in their lives, and that specialness they felt in sharing news with you has in a sense been violated. Imagine how you would feel if your children freely announced to one and all that Dad's fed up with his boss or that you're miffed at the neighbors. Similarly, your children feel that their schoolwork, their friends, and their activities are matters of their own personal concern that can be discussed with you — but are not necessarily for general public consumption.

You must respect these feelings if you want your children to communicate openly with you. You can avoid their exasperation and anger by saying, "Do you mind if I tell Helen what you were telling me about the new friends you made in school?" In this way, you would be respecting their privacy and their dignity, and showing them how to deal with information of a family nature without causing embarrassment.

❦

Moving to the City

Since our children have been babies, we've lived in the suburbs, but now we're about to move to the city because of new job duties my husband has assumed. I'm upset about this. I'm fearful of the more sophisticated urban environment our children will now be in, and I'm wondering if there are ways to cushion them from the shock of being exposed to so many different kinds of people and experiences. I'm also now wondering whether they'll be able to adapt to a school within the city in which the students and teachers are from cultures and backgrounds that are so unfamiliar to our children. What do you think about this?

It sounds to me as if you are far more upset about the situation than you need to be — and your apprehension undoubtedly will be sensed by your children and cause them to feel similarly. I don't mean to imply that a family move is an everyday matter or that it isn't disruptive. But disquieting experiences frequently turn out to be positive ones that can lead to adventure, excitement, and growth.

Unquestionably, your family will need to readjust to a new environment, but making this adjustment will teach your children how to adapt to different people and ways of living. Everyone, I believe, needs to learn these skills in order to cope with the multitude of differences in human nature and cultural backgrounds, and the variety of demands that life places on us.

Children who have been brought up in a "homogenized" environment where everything is simple and predictable miss the excitement of exchanging customs with people from different cultures.

Your move, therefore, can broaden your children's outlook on life — but whether or not this happens depends on how you handle your own feelings about it. If you see this move as an event that has great potential for growth, you'll be better able to cope with some of the inevitable problems that accompany a family move. You will also be better able to help your children see it in a positive way and to deal with some of the problems they'll encounter. Let them know that things will be different and that it will be sad to move away from the places and things with which they've become familiar, but remind them that they can come back from time to time to visit old friends and see their old neighborhood. The move need not be seen as a complete rupture from the past.

At the same time, assure them that they'll make new friends and will adjust to a different school environment. Tell them that you will help them with any problems that they may have, and be willing to talk to their teachers if they have difficulty integrating into the new school. Arouse their enthusiasm about the move by finding out about the special things one can do and see in the city. In New York City, where I live, for example, there are frequent street festivals where people get together to eat the food, play the music, and wear the costumes of different nationalities. On weekends, a child can watch mimes and clowns perform, and can hear musicians perform in the park. Needless to say, city museums, art galleries, and theater for children provide stimulation and learning experiences that are hard to match in a small community.

If you can handle this transition as a family, sharing both the problems and the newfound pleasures, it will serve to solidify your family unity and prepare you to take on whatever challenges you and your family will meet in the future.

Explaining a Stroke

My children constantly play with their friends who live in a neighboring house. Recently, the grandfather of those children came to live with them. He had recently suffered a stroke, and although he is obviously a kind man, he seems "strange" to my children because of his unnatural speech and inability to move about easily. My five-year-old is frightened and runs away when he sees the man, and my seven-year-old asked me in a concerned voice if he "would be like that someday." Should I pretend there's nothing the matter? Or should I try to explain to the children? What do I say?

Explain to your children that a stroke happens when a blood clot blocks the flow of blood to the brain and damages it. Tell them that it can impair a person's ability to speak or walk. Some people completely recover from their strokes; others can only partially recover. Point out to them that even if people who have had strokes can't speak, they probably can hear and may understand everything that is going on around them. Don't hesitate to arouse their compassion for a stroke victim by pointing out how difficult it is for that person, and suggest that it would be nice for them to speak to their neighbor, smile at him, and express a feeling of friendship or warmth. Acknowledge that the man may look strange to them and that this strangeness can be a little scary. Assure them, however, that their friend's grandfather is not trying to be scary, but that he can't help it. While you won't be able to allay all their anxieties and concerns — and you needn't feel you have to — you'll help them develop a feeling of acceptance and compassion for those human differences that are handicapping to some people. I see nothing wrong with responding to your child's question, "Will I be like that someday?" by saying that it's possible for such a thing to happen to anyone, but that young people rarely suffer strokes, and it only happens to some older people. I don't believe we should shield children from facing all of life's unpleasant realities as long as we help the children to understand and cope with their reality.

❦

Rebelling Against Parents' Religion

Religious observances have always been at the heart of our family's holiday celebrations. But this year, for the first time, our fifteen-year-old son says he refuses to come to Midnight Mass with us — he says he "doesn't believe any of that stuff any more" and wants no part of it. We're heartbroken and don't know how to handle this. Should we take a strong moral stand and insist that he come? And how should we explain our son's conduct to our younger children? I'm so afraid this is going to ruin our whole day.

It's not uncommon for young people to depart from the religious beliefs of their parents at some time. But a very large percentage of these young people do resume their family's traditions and beliefs at a later time.

There's no way you can force your child to accept ideas he's rejected. In all likelihood, the more pressure you put upon him, the greater will be his resistance. If you take a strong or punitive stand about all this, and try to frighten him into accepting your views, you may indeed get him to accompany you on this occasion, but your gain may be short term only.

Let him know how important participating in holiday celebrations has been to you and that all your memories of the past are very pleasant ones. Explain that you are disappointed that he does not want to unite with the family in the holiday traditions and that you hope he will reconsider his decision and join in. From your point of view, it would be ideal if he were genuinely committed to your beliefs. But while I'm not suggesting that you compromise your moral position, I'd say you'd gain much more in the long run if you suggested that he participate simply as a matter of tradition. I believe that your relaxed and accepting attitude will do much more to bring him around to your faith than any evangelical lectures will ever do. The warm family feeling and the pleasantness of the holiday atmosphere is often enough to keep alive some of the spirituality you've so diligently tried to transmit to your son.

Let your younger children know that you are somewhat disappointed but that you will not try to force any of your children to accept your beliefs, even though your sincere desire is to have them follow and maintain the faith and the traditions of the family. Let them know that although you hope that they will continue to share these experiences with you as they get older, at some time as they grow up, their feelings may also change. I'm convinced that the more options you give your children and the greater freedom they are allowed to believe what they want, the more likely they will be to follow in your footsteps. I don't think you should be shocked or horrified or take a very self-righteous position, for this might serve to alienate children even more. The more pleasant and gratifying family religious experiences are, the more likely young people will be to maintain and embrace the spirit behind them.

❦

Developing Respect for All Faiths

In school, our seven-year-old has been learning about how people in other countries celebrate the holidays. For the first time she's beginning to realize that all people don't believe in the same things that she's been taught, about God and Mary and Joseph and baby Jesus. My husband and I have a deep commitment to our own religion, and we definitely want our child to share that — yet we also want her to respect the spiritual beliefs of others. How do you explain to a child that "other people believe other things" without undermining the principles of your own faith?

Most seven-year-olds, your own included, are aware of the fact that people are different from one another in the way they look, the way they think, and the way they behave — and in the beliefs they have. It would not only be dishonest and misleading but would threaten your own credibility if you led your children to believe that all people share your own religious beliefs. For this reason, you have to realistically acknowledge the beliefs of others and show by example how you respect other people whose ideas and customs are different from your own.

I'm sure that respect for others is well within the principles of your own religious philosophy. Let your daughter know how strongly you feel about your religion, and point out that other people feel similarly about theirs. In no way are you undermining your own faith by acknowledging the faiths of others. In fact, you are illustrating by example the principles of love and compassion on which most religions are based.

As far as school is concerned, my own personal preference is that children be taught that even though people throughout the world may have different ways of worship, at this time of the year they generally celebrate in a similar manner. They exchange gifts; they sing, dance, and feast. Some schools call their holiday celebrations "year-end celebrations" rather than ascribe what they do to any one particular religious group. When children are aware and accepting of the beliefs of others, they feel a greater unity with all people everywhere. They can experience for themselves the peace and goodwill that is the true spirit of the holiday season.

Feeling Guilty

My fifteen-year-old has said she doesn't want to come along on our regular visits to see her grandfather in a nursing home. When I've insisted, she told me that I'm "just trying to make her feel guilty." Is she right? I hear so much about guilt lately, and I'm confused. Aren't there circumstances when people should feel guilty? How should I handle this situation?

Make it clear to your daughter that it is her *own* conscience that is making her feel guilty, not any pressure on your part. Obviously, she has a sense of "right" and "wrong" — and if she herself didn't feel that her refusal to visit her grandfather was wrong, then she wouldn't feel the least bit guilty. By blaming you for her discomfort, she doesn't have to face her own guilty conscience and cope with the feelings it arouses.

It is fine to acknowledge your daughter's feelings and let her know that you understand that such a visit can seem boring, unpleasant, or depressing to her. But talk with her about the fact that these visits bring joy and happiness into her grandfather's life and that you feel a sense of responsibility toward him and want him to know he is still a part of a loving family.

I believe that guilt can be a very positive force in life. It serves as a guide to reinforce behavior that is socially acceptable and helpful to other people; when people act in ways that are unkind or destructive, a healthy sense of guilt causes them to reevaluate their behavior and act in ways that are more considerate and generous in the future. Unfortunately, there are some people who, because of the circumstances in their early lives, never develop a conscience or a concept of "right" and "wrong." These people commit antisocial acts without any remorse whatsoever, acting out any impulse without regard for its effect on others. They seem to have no sense of guilt about harming other people or destroying property, and their only discomfort may come from a fear of getting caught. While guilt is an unpleasant emotion, it is an important one, and one that helps keep our society organized and people acting toward each other in fair and civilized ways.

I don't mean to say that at *any* time anyone feels guilty, the guilt is positive or psychologically appropriate. Some people feel guilty about *everything*, even their mere existence, and whenever anything goes wrong, they react as though they are personally responsible. This kind of ever-present and inappropriate guilt reflects underlying emotional disturbances and requires professional psychological help to reduce its unpleasantness and bring it into a more healthy focus.

❦

Parental Over-Control

I am a thirty-five-year-old woman, and the mother of two, and my mother still makes me feel guilty if I don't talk to her and fuss over her every few days. She acts very hurt that I don't call more often, and even says that I must not love her since I pay so little attention to her. I do love my mother — so her accusations confuse and depress me, and I feel terrible for hours after our conversations. Can you give me some insight into what's happening? How should I handle this situation?

It sounds to me as if your mother is trying to control your behavior. She first elicits your sympathy and then turns it into guilt because you have supposedly neglected her and failed to shower her with attention. In all likelihood the guilt you feel toward her is not due to a lack of genuine love on your part but grows out of the anger she arouses because she is trying to control your emotions. If you feel content with the amount of attention you show her and have a sincere feeling of affection for her, then make it clear that you love her but cannot be completely responsible for her unhappiness. Explain that you get angry and annoyed when she insists otherwise.

Some parents are very, very manipulative and try to control their children by playing on their emotions and arousing guilt in unfair ways. In all likelihood, at various times in your life, she has consciously or unconsciously "made you feel guilty" to get you to act in the ways she wanted — and now a frustrating pattern has been established. The more you allow yourself to be manipulated, the more you encourage this to continue.

I see no reason why you can't set your mother straight by pointing out that you do indeed care about her happiness and will do whatever you reasonably can to help her make new friends and develop new interests. But the responsibility for her happiness is not totally up to you, and she must take steps herself to fill her time with projects and activities that are rewarding.

❧

Blaming Children Unfairly

Whenever my sister's young children disappoint her — by getting poor grades in school or getting into mischief — she tells them they "make Mommy unhappy." Since my sister tends to be chronically depressed anyway, I think this is a terrible thing to say to children. Isn't it possible the children will think they are the cause of her unhappiness? Should parents ever say such things?

There's nothing wrong with parents letting children know that their misbehavior causes unhappiness or discomfort. This helps children realize that their behavior does indeed have an effect on other people. If parents avoid showing feelings about how their children act, children will, in all likelihood, think that "my parents don't care" and have no standards or values on which to model their own behavior.

On the other hand, it is certainly wrong for children to get the idea that they are responsible for all of their parents' feelings. That unquestionably puts an unfair burden on children and can be destructive in their lives. If a parent is indeed going through an obvious and prolonged period of anger or depression due to other personal problems, he or she should make it clear to children that they are not the sole cause of the upset.

It is natural that children who get poor grades in school should cause a parent some consternation. But don't let it stop there. Explain to your children that you are sure they too are unhappy about their poor grades, and would be very proud of themselves if they worked harder to improve. In this way a parent's emotional reactions help guide children and at the same time instill in them a sense of personal responsibility for their own emotional well-being.

I would like to add that it's always important to bear in mind that children who get into mischief repeatedly and do poorly in school may be *trying* to get a reaction from their parents — and in this case they do it by behaving in a negative way. My experience tells me that when this occurs, parents usually have failed to give their children the positive recognition and attention they needed in their day-to-day lives, and probably have ignored them except when they got into trouble.

There's nothing wrong with letting children know, from time to time, that they cause parental unhappiness. But you must also point out with equal vigor the happiness, pride, and joy they bring into your life with their achievements, satisfactions, and cooperation.

❧

Parental Drinking Problem

My husband has been working under a great deal of pressure lately and has been drinking very heavily. He gets so irritable — sometimes even violent — that we don't know how to deal with him. My children seem anxious and nervous. Should I talk to my husband, or should I ignore the problem and assume it will go away? What should I say to the children?

It's essential that you talk both to your husband and your children about the problem. Explain to your children that their father has been under a great deal of pressure and that it's not unusual for people overwhelmed by stress to drink more in an attempt to relax and forget their problems. Explain that while liquor often provides temporary relief, it never provides any real solution, and only leads to heavier drinking when the problems don't go away. You can say these things without in any way making their father look foolish for his attempts to ease his pain; and if you explain that his outbursts of rage are a direct result of the alcohol's effect on his personality, they'll understand further that it is the alcohol that's at fault, not their father. Let your children know that their own nervousness and anxiety are completely understandable; after all, they're not seeing the father they're used to. Point out that the problem is nothing to be ashamed or afraid of, but that it will take the support and understanding of everyone in the family to help overcome it.

Unfortunately, it's very difficult to get a person with a drinking problem to accept help; first he must accept the reality of the problem, then the severity of it. Approach your husband directly, lovingly — without the children, as that would be embarrassing for him and for them — when he hasn't been drinking and when he seems calm. Most important is for you to understand that your husband's problem is an illness, one that can be treated, so that you in no way use an accusing or belittling tone. It's essential that he feel your support and love, that he know you're aware of the terrible stress he feels and the feelings of inadequacy it can cause. Make him understand your concern now is not only for him but for the family; tell him you know he loves his children but that it can't get through to them when he is drinking, and that the effects on them could be devastating and irreparable if he doesn't stop. Assure him that you and the children respect and trust him and that in no way will your faith in him be interrupted if he will acknowledge the problem and accept help.

❦

Explaining Heart Attacks

My father was a healthy man all his life. Suddenly, at the age of sixty-seven, he had a heart attack. Should we tell our young children about their grandfather's illness, or will that make them worry unnecessarily about the possibility that this could happen to them?

Hiding the truth by pretending nothing has happened to your father will only damage your children's trust in you. If you withhold vital information from them, they'll simply seek out other people as their source, and others may not be as accurate or as gentle as you would be. Moreover, when children feel alienated from the family, it's difficult for them to feel secure about their parents' love. After all, if you're not honest with them about some important facts, why should they believe you when you tell them others — like that you love them?

Explain to your children what a heart attack is; say that we know to a certain extent why people get them, that children almost never get them, and that they often can be prevented.

That way you'll very quickly establish that they needn't worry about getting Grandpa's illness now and that they have some control over whether they get it later, as well.

If your children are worried about the well-being of their grandfather, however, their concern is perfectly appropriate, and you should express your own worry about him as well. Reassure them, though, that he is getting excellent medical care, that he is comfortable, and that with proper rest it is possible he will recover and live a long life. Explain that no one knows how much damage was done, but that when a person survives a heart attack, he often takes much better care of himself than he used to and may get much healthier than he used to be as a result. Don't worry too much about your children's concern about their grandfather; sickness is a very real part of life, and hiding it makes it more frightening than it need be. Moreover, a little worry might help your children really see the importance of taking good care of themselves throughout their lives.

❦

Making the Family Move Easier

While a family move isn't the greatest tragedy in the world, for us at the moment it seems to be. We have to move or my husband will lose an excellent job. My children are in tears because they don't want to leave this community where they've always lived and where all their friends are. How can we make this move easier for them?

Tell your children that most of the warmth, love, and security you all feel as a family comes from sharing not only pleasures but the crises as well. Explain that if you had your way, this move would not take place; but since it is going to happen, that you're going to do everything within your power to make it pleasant. Perhaps you could begin to stress the adventure inherent in the move — that while it may seem scary now, the new friends they'll make and the new opportunities they'll have will be very exciting. I don't think you'd be overdramatizing things by pointing out that throughout history, Americans frequently moved in order to seek better opportunities and explore new frontiers. Let them know that the pioneers also had mixed feelings — they looked, hoped, and wished for a more full life, but at the same time they were frightened, anxious, and aware that things might not always work out the way they wanted.

Sometimes it's wise to take the children to the new community prior to the actual move, to visit the school, meet neighbors, and just get some impression of where they're going. That alone is often enough to get the children a little bit excited about their new lives. At the least, it replaces the unknown with a welcome reality that they usually appreciate.

❦

The Ailing, Depressed Grandmother

My grandmother was always lively and full of life and could do as many things as she liked. Lately though, since she's had trouble with arthritis and an assortment of other ailments, we've tried to get her to take it easy; and even though we do everything we can to wait on her, she seems very depressed. Is this sort of personality change natural? How should we handle it?

Unfortunately, your grandmother's depression is a very common occurrence in older people. Doctors sometimes describe it as involutional melancholia because it is a depression that results from physical changes that take place in the course of the aging process.

To a great extent your grandmother is probably reacting to the fact that she is no longer able to do all the things she enjoyed before. I'm sure she recognizes this, is in part angry and frustrated by it, and feels helpless in not being able to cope with things she used to take in her stride. And when others wait on her and "help her do things," it simply emphasizes all the more her increasing helplessness and isolation.

While it is probably necessary to give her some assistance, do everything you can to encourage her to use her own resources, and offer as much stimulation as you can in her life. Try to get her to visit friends or have her entertain them at home. While she may not be able to walk the distances she once did, encourage her to get out and take short walks and carry on with as many activities as she can. As much as possible, help her maintain her independence and dignity. Above all, give her a sense of importance as a member of your family and a person in your life.

❧

Grief at Death of a Pet

Our family dog was struck by a car and killed. Of course we all were very sad, but our ten-year-old daughter took it especially hard. It's been a week now, and she still seems upset and cries about "poor Sandy." Is it natural for a chid to grieve this way? Her twelve-year-old brother felt terrible too, but he seems to have gotten over it.

Yes, it is natural for a child to react this way after the sudden death of a devoted pet. While it is very discomforting for everyone around her to see her reaction, it is a tribute to your child's

215

sensitivity and capacity for deep love, and you should accept her feelings while giving her as much support as you possibly can. Tell her that you understand her feelings and agree that no other pet will ever *really* take the place of Sandy — but at the same time you want to think about getting another family dog and would like her to help choose the new pet.

Your son's resolution of the dog's death in a shorter period of time does not mean he is either braver or less sensitive, it simply means he had less of a tie to the dog or is simply different in temperament.

❦

Adult Mood Swings

I have mood swings that seem to hit for no apparent reason. Things will seem fine and then all of a sudden I'll be plunged into low-grade grumpiness or real despair. My daughter says this could be due to some chemical imbalance. Is this possible, or is it all due to emotional factors?

Such fluctuating mood swings definitely can be caused by a chemical or hormonal imbalance. In recent years doctors have treated this kind of depression at its source and have obtained dramatic results by administering drugs to correct this imbalance and restore a patient's sense of well-being.

Unquestionably, factors in a person's past, or problems in the present, also play a part; if and when a chemical imbalance exists, it is simply harder to deal with emotional stress. At various times, if you are physiologically predisposed to feeling "blue," then your reactions can be intensified by attitudes or conflicts from the past or problems in the present. For example, following childbirth there is an abrupt change in the balance of hormones in a woman's body, which can make her vulnerable to postpartum depression. If a woman has mixed feelings about being a parent, her physical state in a sense sets her up (or brings her down) so that her emotional reactions are intensified.

It is extremely important for you to have a medical check-up. Be sure to give your doctor a very careful, detailed history of when these mood swings take place and what seems to trigger them. From there, your doctor can proceed with tests to determine more about the nature of your depressions and how they should be treated.

❦

Grin and Wear It — It's the Thought That Counts

I was touched that my eight-year-old daughter and ten-year-old son had saved their allowances to buy me a birthday gift, but when I opened the box and discovered a fluorescent purple shirt decorated with yellow birds, I was a little taken aback. I thanked the children profusely — and now they're asking me when I'll be wearing the shirt. Should I wear it, even though I look ridiculous in it?

Grin and wear it — it's the thought that counts and not the gift. Your children exercised their best judgment and, in all likelihood, went to great trouble to please you. Their efforts, and the love it represents, are the greatest birthday gift you could have received. If you look at it in this way, you'll realize that your finickiness about fashion is not nearly as important as the sincerity of their gesture. Wear the shirt proudly, especially in their company — and if you feel it's necessary, simply announce to everyone who sees you that "this is a gift from my children."

Perhaps if something like this happens again in the future, and you really don't think you can bring yourself to wear the gift, you can express your enthusiasm by saying, "How wonderfully thoughtful of you to buy me a shirt — it's something I need and like very much. But I wonder if I might exchange it for one that goes with a special outfit I have in mind?" In this way you will be expressing your appreciation and acknowledging your children's values. At the same time, you will be adapting their gift to one that better fits your own taste and lifestyle.

Index